Intermittent Fasting for Women:

The Complete Beginner's Guide for Weight Loss Burn Fat—Heal Your Body Through the Special Intermittent Process, and Live a Healthy Lifestyle

Table of Contents

Introduction 1

Chapter 1: What Is Intermittent Fasting? 3
    A Quick History Lesson About Fasting and Intermittent Fasting 14

Chapter 2: Incredible Benefits of Intermittent Fasting 16

Chapter 3: The Various Types and Methods of Intermittent Fasting 29
    Types of Intermittent Fasting 30
    How to Find Your Personal Intermittent Fasting Method 39

Chapter 4: Secret Techniques for Feasting on Your Favorite Foods 47

Chapter 5: Tips and Tricks for Staying Motivated While Intermittent Fasting 61

Chapter 6: How Fasting Works to Safely Increase Weight Loss .. 76
    All About Ketosis 85

Chapter 7: The Process of Autophagy and Why It Is So Important for Women 92
    More on the Science of Autophagy and Women 100

Chapter 8: Intermittent Fasting for Women 107

Chapter 9: How to Start Intermittent Fasting 117

Chapter 10: Common Mistakes While Fasting and How to Avoid Them 128

Conclusion 140

Introduction

Thank you for downloading *Intermittent Fasting for Women: The Complete Beginner's Guide for Weight Loss—Burn Fat, Heal Your Body Through the Special Intermittent Process, and Live a Healthy Lifestyle*, and congratulations on doing so!

Throughout this book, you will pass through chapter after chapter of a discussion on intermittent fasting and how it applies to women specifically. You will encounter a good dose of medical references and resources, but also a lot of applicable tips and techniques for making this eating plan a reality for your life. There are some dangers to consider when adjusting your food intake, but there are some amazing benefits to consider as well. Follow the suggestions in this book for advice on how to implement an intermittent fast safely and more realistically into your daily life, with the intention of it lasting for a long time. The content of this book is mainly presented for how intermittent fasting applies to the female gender; however, there are many concepts that can be applied to men as well. Just ignore the discussion on menopause and ovaries in that case!

Whenever you consider making a drastic change to the way you eat and drink, you need to make sure you are making an informed decision. You need to understand the foundation of the concept and why it is a healthy and real plan that will make a difference in your life. This is why you will find links to scholarly articles outlining in more detail (and more scientific language) the findings of intermittent fasting on animals and humans in relationship to everything from losing weight to treating asthma. This means, if you want to dive in further into the scientific side of things, you have a good place to start from. Many of the articles referenced in the book were referenced as the foundation for the concepts and advice in the chapters. The goal is to give you the information so you can make a good decision for yourself.

There are plenty of books on this subject on the market, so thanks again for choosing this one! Every effort was made to ensure it is full of as much useful information as possible. Please enjoy!

Chapter 1: What Is Intermittent Fasting?

Now is the time to fast, ladies! Thanks to the publications in Good Housekeeping, Women's Health, and the BBC, this diet trend has created an increased interest in this "latest" trend. Ready to give it a shot? One thing you may not have read much about is that this trend is actually not new. Fasting has been occurring for thousands of years. This raises the questions about what fasting really is, why people should consider it, and how to do it safely. When beginning the exploration process, it can seem daunting or overwhelming to ponder these questions. Often, people do not know where to start for sustained benefits. If this is you, do not worry—that is the purpose of this book! The definition found in the Merriam-Webster dictionary explains fasting as "to eat sparingly and abstain from certain foods" and "to abstain from food". This basic definition begins to reveal, and also confuse, exactly what fasting looks like for modern people. According to this definition, all you need to do is stop eating food, stop eating a certain amount of food, or just cut certain foods out. If this answers the first question of what fasting is, the next question to consider is why should people consider fasting. Is there a valid reason to restrict your body of its fuel source?

Fasting is chosen for a variety of reasons, being health as the primary reason, then weight management and religion. The purpose for religious fasting and the foundational principles for following the religious fasting regimen are well-established, and if you have chosen to fast for religious purposes, chances are you already understand these. For the purposes of this book, religious fasting will not be covered in depth. This leaves two additional reasons for fasting: health and weight management. What may surprise you is that you are probably already following a form of fasting. A lot of advice is thrown out in the nutrition and fitness industry about not eating a meal after 7 PM, drinking a lot of water, and then eating a good breakfast after 7 AM. What often follows this advice does not always expand on the reason for doing this. One of the best reasons is to prevent you from going to bed with a full stomach. This allows the digestive system to rest as well, resulting in less gas and indigestion waking the body during the night. In addition, sleeping is a calming state, which means the body does not engage in much or any physical exercise. If you have a lot of food in the stomach when entering into this sustained restful state, the body does not burn off the calories taken in, meaning the food is then changed into fat that is stored in the body. The benefits for following this advice are giving your body the opportunity to store calories for more active parts of the day, encourages a better night's sleep, and allows the body to fully rest. Not many people share this information when telling you to not grab that second helping once 7 PM hits.

Weight management and weight loss are the third reason for fasting; it is also connected with the health goals mentioned above. Fasting has gained popularity in the mainstream media mainly for this benefit: it can help you lose weight and keep it off. Weight loss is the reason for the "rediscovery" of this dieting method. Similar to how to the Paleo or "Caveman" diet is revisiting the older methods for eating food, fasting is mimicking how people used to have to wait to eat their next meal. Sometimes, this waiting lasted for days. This is why the body stores fat for stretches of time between meals when the body needs energy. Fasting today means tricking the body into thinking it needs to open up the fat storage to fuel the body because the food is "scarce". The benefit of doing this from a weight perspective is that this method does not lower bloating by cutting back on sodium intake or help you drop quick pounds from water retention, but rather reaches into the "stubborn" fat pockets that hold on to fat like a life raft. This sounds like an ideal situation, but now it leads to the next question of what is the best way to burn that stubborn fat, to improve overall health, and to lose a couple inches around the waistline.

Fasting comes in a variety of forms. Depending on your goals, personality, and health needs, fasting can last for a few days with no food or water or a few hours with restricted foods. Most of the time, the physicians, before medical procedures, recommend a "full" fast. There are multiple benefits for completing this type of fast for this reason, but it is one of the most accessible examples of a full fast application. Religious fasts can also follow a strict full fast regimen. The body needs water for survival, so this type of fast should always be approached with caution. These fasts should never last longer than three days. Another type of fasting is called a "regular" fast. It is similar to a full fast but does allow for water consumption. Because participants can drink water during this fast, it can be adhered to for long stretches of time without severely endangering most people's health.

Recall back to the definition of fasting from the dictionary, particularly the part about abstaining from some foods. An example of a type of fasting that embodies this definition is the "partial" fast. This type of fasting deals in the types of foods and drinks that are consumed. Sometimes, a "partial" fast is recommended to someone who suspects a food allergy or sensitivity. This fast is adhered to for a certain number of days to allow the body to remove the traces of the suspected food, and the person is observed to see if their symptoms improve. Then, the food is reintroduced, again for observational reasons, noticing if the body shows signs of a reaction. For people looking to "ease" into fasting, this is a good method of starting a change, especially if major changes have failed or never been attempted before. Some of the common foods people begin cutting out include fast foods, processed foods, soda, and candy. This Partial fast lasts for a few days to a couple weeks. Once successful in removing these foods, the person can add foods to the list to cut out for a longer time frame. This is good to remember as you begin to dive further into the next type of fasting, and the topic of this book, "intermittent" fasting.

An intermittent fast is like a combination of a regular fast and a partial fast. It combines the removal of food except for water or a restriction of caloric intake for a certain time frame. There are many different variations of this fasting method which will be explained further in this book, but it is helpful to remember the example of not eating after 7 PM shared earlier in this chapter. This is an example of an intermittent fast. A person cuts out food for a span of a few hours or severely limits the amount of food they eat in that time frame. Sometimes, the limitations last for 24 hours but followed by a structured time for eating and then fasting, such as one-day fasting, then one-day free eating followed by the next day of fasting. During Ramadan, the Muslim community is encouraged to follow a form of intermittent fasting, only eating during the darkness, and abstaining from food during daylight hours.

Part of the allure of this type of fasting is that you are not cutting foods out forever. For example, if you are craving a donut, you do not have to lament over the fact that you can never eat donuts again. Instead, you can erase the knowledge that you are choosing not to eat the donut today or before 7 AM, but the next morning or once the clock turns 7:01 AM, you can indulge in that sweet treat. This method is also a flexible method, meaning you can ease into it, similar to the benefits of doing a partial fast. For example, you can choose to fast for one day of the week, making no other dietary changes to the rest of the days in the week. This fasting method also does not need to last a full 24 hours. Some people choose to fast for twelve hours of the day or just cut out certain foods on a certain day. For example, enjoying "Fish Friday" or "Meatless Monday" are examples of a type of intermittent fasting, helping you ease into fasting.

It is interesting to note that in many observations and experiences, when people participate in intermittent fasting, they begin to make different and often healthier choices on the days that they are not fasting. It is a great relief to many that on the days when they are not fasting, they can enjoy whatever foods they want and in whatever quantities they desire. But after a while, the body begins to reject those foods in favor of healthier options, which adds another benefit to following an intermittent fasting plan. Part of the reason for this is because of the natural instinct of your brain for survival as well as the recognition that sometimes you are "bored hungry," "emotionally hungry," or actually hungry.

True hunger is a subtle sensation that you begin to understand while on intermittent fasting. When you can recognize this feeling in relation to the other feelings, you can help your body cut off cravings and mitigate overeating habits. Additionally, a chemical is released during an intermittent fast, alerting the brain and the body that it needs to self-regulate and not rely on incoming nutrients. This chemical is essential for helping balance hunger habits and weight management. These processes, however, are not immediate. Like all good health and wellness plans that have the added benefit of weight loss and management, the process takes time to show the results of the hard work.

Many practitioners suggest following an intermittent fasting plan for about two weeks to challenge your body and also allow your body to show a few changes. But during this time, it is important to also recognize that the body may not readily accept the new changes to its fuel intake. For example, it is common for people to experience some digestion issues or minor gut irritations. Other common side effects include withdrawal symptoms, such as headaches or irritability. These symptoms are related to your body adjusting to its more instinctual functioning and the switch from food-for-fuel to fat-for-fuel taking place. When you start this process, make sure to spend time observing your body. Be gracious to yourself as the demands of your body change during this introductory phase. As the weeks continue, hopefully, you will notice that your cravings for junk foods or high-calorie foods will begin to diminish. Also, ideally you will notice the discomfort during fasting periods begin to subside. But, like typical health plans, it is important to also examine concerns and implementation strategies for best results.

When you begin to consider the concerns of adopting a new lifestyle and are wondering how to safely implement it into daily life, rest assured that you are in the correct frame of mind. Approaching intermittent fasting as an individual experience is important. Intermittent fasting impacts the health of the individual. It can make positive changes but also has the potential to negatively impact as well. For example, if you have previously struggled with an eating disorder in the past, fasting without direct medical supervision is not recommended. The purpose of intermittent fasting is to improve health and well-being, not to cause harm. Also, those with diabetes should exercise caution with intermittent fasting. People with diabetes need to maintain a healthy level of glucose and the body naturally fluctuates during fasting periods. This fluctuation can be dangerous if not under medical supervision. These health complications defeat the purpose of intermittent fasting. An additional concern is for women who are pregnant. Infants and pregnant women require certain levels of vitamins and calories for optimal health, and intermittent fasting can cause unnecessary harm. Other concerns for individuals who are overweight and of healthy weight are examined further in this book.

Now that you are aware of some of the medical conditions that need medical supervision while participating in intermittent fasting, you can decide if it is the right time to start this diet plan and how it will fit into your life. Most of the health conditions outlined above already require consistent doctor visits. Bringing up your interest in this diet plan on your next visit is a great place to start. If you do not have one of those medical concerns, are looking to improve your general health, and are also interested in losing weight, it is best to start by examining personal and lifestyle habits. For example, do you recognize that you have trouble keeping commitments to yourself and others? Have you been able to remove something from your life in the past with ease or minimal discomfort? It is also important to consider your success or challenges with dieting in the past. Did you struggle to get past the first few days of a diet or were you able to complete a cleanse or several-week diet plan in the past easily? If you notice that you struggle with dieting and commitments, it is probably best to begin a few steps at a time. This might look like implementing something like a "Fish Friday" to start. For others, it might look like a day without soda or processed foods. It can be for a twelve-hour time span or a full 24 hours. After choosing a reasonable place to start, try it out for a few weeks to see how you do. Once you successfully follow a plan for two weeks in a row, consider increasing the commitment. This may look like more time abstaining from a specific food or more foods are cut away. Continue to gradually increase from the starting point. For others that have had more success with making modifications in the past, a good starting point is to choose one day during the week to abstain from food for 12 hours. This could be during the day or overnight or can be a complete abstention from food or partial. Additional tips on how to implement and follow intermittent fasting for the best success will be shared later on for you as well. Hopefully, this gives you a good idea of where to begin and how customized you can make it fit into your life.

A Quick History Lesson About Fasting and Intermittent Fasting

Throughout the world, fasting has been a go-to remedy for a number of healing functions for thousands of years. In fact, Hippocrates often prescribed fasting and intermittent fasting to help "starve" an illness. Later, Plutarch, another ancient Greek, encouraged his readers to fast for health instead of reaching for medicines. Later, other great thought leaders, including Aristotle and Plato, supported fasting as a way to heal the body. Like most animals, humans naturally refuse food when they are sick. This is an instinctual process for healing the body from the inside. This "instinct" reveals that fasting for health has been around as long as humankind and is a way to help support and find optimal health for the body.

In addition to health, it was believed that intermittent fasting also improved mental capacity. By allowing the blood to flow to the brain and other vital organs, instead of to the GI tract during periods of digestion, mental awareness is improved. One of the "fathers" of Western medicine and the founder of toxicology, Philip Paracelsus, wrote that fasting was a way of invoking the "physician within". Benjamin Franklin, a renowned founding father, and intellect, also wrote: "The best of all medicines is resting and fasting." Today, fasting and intermittent fasting is still being used as a means for healing and helping the body find homeostasis, as well as the myriad of other benefits it brings.

Chapter 2: Incredible Benefits of Intermittent Fasting

Changing lifestyle and diet usually occurs when a person decides to live a healthier life. The "right" choices for their body and to feel good are typically the driving force. Honestly reflect on your own preference; either you want to feel energized and healthy or fatigued and sick. Most likely, you chose the first option! The choice to be healthier is made to minimize or cure pre-existing health conditions or to prevent a disease from occurring. This can be summarized as either restorative or preventative reasons. A major part of the healing and healthy process involves the diet, no matter what reason a person has for making a change. The link between diet and cancer is highlighted on the American Cancer Society's webpage, for example. Exercise and diet are two improvements people can make to their lifestyle to prevent most forms of cancer from developing and spreading. One of the answers to the question of a healthy lifestyle, especially for women, is intermittent fasting. Women tend to respond quicker to the gene associated with the feeling of hunger while men tend to take a little longer to biologically react.

One of the scariest moments of a person's life can occur when a doctor sits you down in their office and explains that you have cancer. Even thinking about hearing this news can cause people to stop what they are doing and consider a different path. Cervical and breast cancers are two types of cancer that are unique to women. This adds additional stress and fear for women and cancer.

Cancer cells are known for growth and rapid spreading. One way to prevent cancer is to stop or slow down this process, which is where fasting comes in.

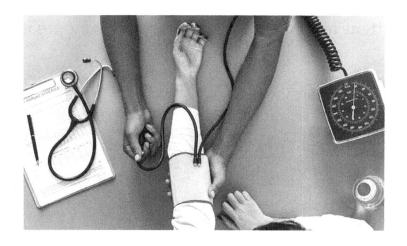

Fasting can help stunt the progression of cancer cells, ultimately preventing them from getting to where they want to go. This is done through new blood deprivation during fasting periods. This weakens or cripples the cells, making them more vulnerable to additional treatments. Also, in a study conducted on mice with breast cancer, short-term fasting, such as intermittent fasting, showed incredible results in treating the disease. The FDA is also interested in the benefits of intermittent fasting and cancer treatment. In a report published in 2016, the FDA asked patients about their preferred methods for cancer treatment, and it should come as no surprise that diet modification was one of the most popular and utilized methods of treatment while being treated for cancer. At this time the FDA is considering publicizing the benefits of intermittent fasting and cancer prevention and treatment!

Treatment for cancer using intermittent fasting still requires more human studies to definitively say that its "cures" cancer; however, it is very clear that it can help prevent its development in the first place. Adjusting consumed foods on non-fasting days can also help increase prevention and treatment results.

Another disease that affects many people, and is also a scary diagnosis, is diabetes. Sugar in the blood, or glucose, is something that naturally occurs. A "healthy" body is sensitive to this substance and works to remove it so the body remains regulated. But in a person with diabetes, the sensitivity changes and the body either removes too much or too little. This is why people with diabetes have to prick their finger and test their blood, as well as inject insulin into their bloodstream. Maintaining this balance is crucial, and there are ways to help the body remember or develop sensitivity, even if the body has never been sensitive to it before, as is the case for many type 1 diabetics. There have been a number of studies conducted on intermittent fasting and diabetes. In many of the results published, a large majority was able to stop relying on insulin and was able to maintain a healthy blood sugar level. Even people with diabetes from birth saw vast improvements to their treatment of the disease. Note that most of the studies prefaced these findings with alternate fasting plans of 24 hours on and 24 hours off, with participants also being cognizant of their nutrition intake on the days when eating.

Obesity is also often linked to diabetes, type 2 diabetes specifically. When following an intermittent fasting diet plan, many participants see an effective approach for maintaining lean mass while losing and keeping off excess pounds. It is the process of keeping off the weight that is most important to the prevention and treatment of diabetes. This is one of the reasons intermittent fasting is a favorable option; it has a history of keeping the weight away. Women are also more receptive to the positive impacts of intermittent fasting and diabetes.

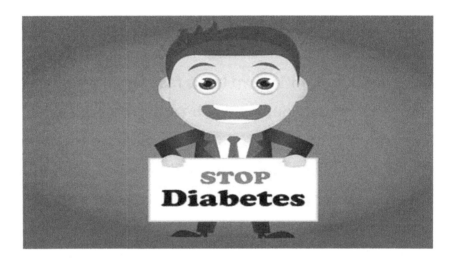

A healthy concern that leads to many other diseases is high blood pressure. Sometimes, people are sensitive to their blood pressure levels, while others do not know that they suffer from this medical issue. When a person is unaware of the condition, it can cause some major problems if no steps are taken to regulate it. Most of the time, a doctor will prescribe medication to treat high blood pressure, but it is not the only method of treatment to consider. Lifestyle changes can drastically lower blood pressure and, by association, also lowers the risk of developing other health issues related to high blood pressure. Medication is necessary for people who suffer from high blood pressure related to kidney problems, but for people with "hypertension" or an unknown cause for the condition, changing diet and exercise habits can make a big difference.

Intermittent fasting is a natural way of lowering and stabilizing blood pressure. Especially for women going through menopause, where high blood pressure is a common side effect, intermittent fasting has the ability to control blood pressure intrinsically and without medications.

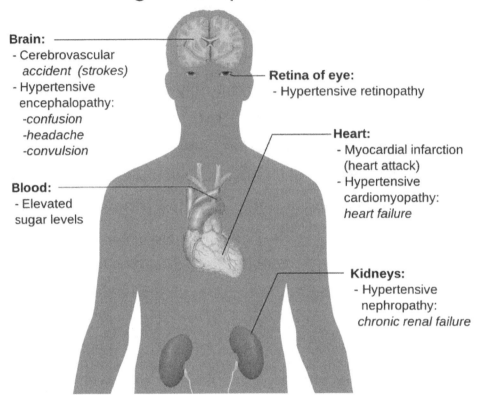

Women experiencing body transitions, such as puberty, pregnancy, and menopause, can often struggle with mental health issues. Depression, anxiety, mood swings, and irritability are common side effects of these transitions. Another common symptom is the instability of emotions. A boost to mental health is positively impacting self-esteem, which can be promoted through fasting and intermittent fasting. For example, when a woman focuses on the "small wins" throughout intermittent fasting, she can feel successful and confident. Also, when the brain reacts to a fasting state, it begins to readjust its mental functioning, impacting states of depression or anxiety positively. The "rewiring" of the brain that takes place during intermittent fasting can also positively impact social interactions, sleep habits, and mood swings. Peace is another common feeling that participants experience while participating in intermittent fasting, which is an uncommon state for people who suffer from various mental health conditions.

Mental health is also impacted by external sources such as societal and peer pressure. Depression can occur when a person feels as if he or she does not belong or doesn't have a support system. Being overweight or obese is not aligned with the Western "idealized figure". This means someone who is or feels that they are overweight can suffer from disconnection and depression. Losing the excess weight can help a person feel more in line with society's norms, allowing them to feel a short-term boost their "tribe acceptance".

An added benefit to improving your health is you also improve the opportunity to live longer! In several medical studies on animals, the test subjects that participated in intermittent fasting habits showed a significant increase in longevity. One of the most promising recent studies was conducted on monkeys, which is often the last animal test subject before human trials begin! It is possible that the life-extending benefits are unique to just intermittent fasting, or it might be because of its proven link to overall health rejuvenation. Some of these known positive impacts include proven cancer prevention, reduction of various disease risks, and increased function of important organs. All of these lead to a longer life as well.

In the study conducted on monkeys, there was a notable difference, not just in the life span of those that followed an intermittent fasting lifestyle, but also between the genders of the monkeys. The male monkeys lived a few years longer than their male counterparts that ate a traditional diet, but the female monkeys following the intermittent fasting schedule lived almost six years longer than their traditional female counterparts! In another study conducted on monkeys, the female monkeys lived almost ten years past their normal life expectancy. It is still in the animal-trial stage, but it is a benefit worth considering!

Following this lifestyle and diet requires a good dose of self-discipline. It can be a challenge and most likely will come with a few tears and a lot of mental conflicts. Of course, any diet and lifestyle change can come with this, but when you are feeling hungry and a tempting commercial comes on TV or a co-worker brings in a big box of hot and fresh donuts, it is your will power that will help you from snacking away the afternoon or into the night. This means that participating in intermittent fasting is both physical and mental. Remember this as you continue down the path.

Emotional eating often shows itself in the form of "real" hunger. As you begin the process, you will be to notice the difference between true hunger and everything else, including thirst. During a fasting stage, when hunger pangs arise, take a moment to identify the feeling and look for the source of the state. Sometimes, this involves giving it the time or a cup of water to see if the feeling passes. If you notice that the feeling is occurring because of boredom or restlessness, look for alternatives to satisfy what is really going on. Common emotional states that often manifest in eating include boredom, stress, anger, or sadness. Instead of reaching for a snack or over-eating at mealtime, becoming aware of the source of the feeling can help you find alternatives to these states. For example, if you are bored, go for a walk or try out a creative hobby. If you are stressed or angry, consider meditation or a punching bag. For those that find they have eaten more than necessary when feeling sad, calling a funny friend or going to see a funny movie can be a good way of dealing with the emotions instead of through eating. Just keep in mind, a good movie in a fun theatre can be awesome, but you will also be surrounded by junk foods and the alluring smell of popcorn. If you love popcorn and a bubbly soda, this could end up being more torture than relief.

Thirst is also commonly shrouded as hunger. The mind can often misinterpret the desire for water as a desire for food, especially something salty! What is interesting is that salt is the opposite of what the body needs in that situation, but the body is weird that way. If you cannot identify an emotional state that is causing your hunger, consider filling up a big cup with water and drink it down slowly. Be observant over the next few minutes and see if your hungry feeling begins to dissipate. After 5 minutes, if you are still feeling hungry, chances are it is true "hunger". If the feeling passes, you have done a good job of identifying the desire for thirst instead of food.

A good mental game you can play with yourself when you are really hungry is to "trick" yourself into thinking it is consuming foods. This is done through a cup of black coffee (no cream or sugar), unsweetened teas, or water flavored with a lemon or lime wedge. The added flavor can make the body feel as if it is consuming food and calories, but it is actually just enjoying a non-caloric drink. These exercises in uncovering the real messages of your body are a great lesson in understanding the needs of your body. This is a major health benefit that can often be overlooked when considering intermittent fasting. In fact, being "tuned in" to the messages being sent and received in your body is one of the best health secrets of this diet and lifestyle and should not be missed. You are learning to hear what your body really needs and finding healthy ways to satisfy its needs and wants.

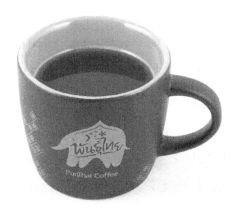

Chapter 3: The Various Types and Methods of Intermittent Fasting

Intermittent fasting is not really a diet plan as much as it is an eating schedule. This method of health balancing and weight stabilizing is not so much about what foods you eat but more about when you eat food. This means you can choose what works realistically with your life and needs and adjust it to fit accordingly and still be part of the intermittent fasting group. When you choose certain times or meals to not eat or to cut back dramatically on caloric intake, you are intentionally selecting times of the day when your body will need to rely on stored energy instead of new, food energy.

Although this can be a highly customizable diet plan for anyone, there are a few methods or types of intermittent fasting people have encouraged in the past. These templates are great places to start or try out when you are finding out how intermittent fasting will fit into your life. Throughout this chapter, you will learn about some of the more common intermittent fasting methods as well as ideas on how to apply it to your life. When you are done with reviewing the various versions, it is advisable to decide which version you would like to adapt to your life and begin formulating a plan. The final part of this chapter will help guide you through this process.

Types of Intermittent Fasting

The first method of intermittent fasting to explore is the 16/8 method. This refers to a span of 8 hours during the day that you plan on eating, leaving the remaining 16 hours of the day for fasting. For some people, this means not eating until lunchtime and then stopping again around 8 PM. Other people enjoy breakfast upon waking and eat an early dinner, about 4 PM. It is possible to adjust the time frame to be shorter or longer, depending on your preference. For those that struggle with making a big commitment, it could be 10 hours of eating with 14 hours of fasting, meaning you eat a later breakfast and lunch leading to normal dinner time, after which you do not eat again until morning. This time frame is also ideal for women, according to recent studies. For biological purposes, women tend to thrive on "shorter" fasting spurts, such as 14 or 15 hours. For those who have seen success after a couple weeks on this method and want to try a different challenge, you can shorten the eating window to 4 or 6 hours, allowing the remaining hours to be dedicated to fasting. The following eating guide is one way to approach this method in your daily life:

Week 1: Begin eating at noon, stop eating at 8 PM.

Week 2: Begin eating at 8 AM, stop eating at 4 PM.

Another way to consider this method is that you are skipping one meal per day. During the first week, you are skipping breakfast, and the second week, you are skipping dinner. Of course, you can also adjust the number of meals you consume in this time frame and can also adjust the times to fit your schedule. For example, if you want to eat at 7 AM, then you would stop eating at 3 PM or if you want to start eating at 11 AM, then you would stop eating at 7 PM. Feel free to move this sliding window to cover any hours of the day that works best for you.

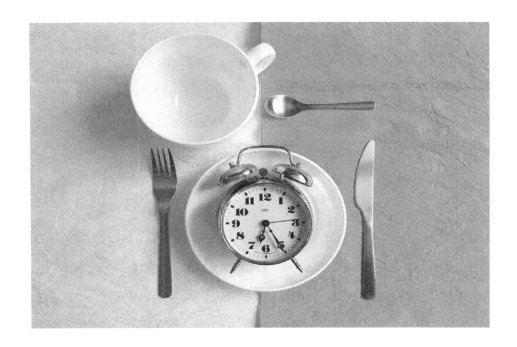

The next intermittent fasting method to consider is the 24-hour fast. This means that after the last meal of the day, you wait until that time the next day to eat again. For example, if you finish dinner at 7 PM, you would not eat anything the next day until 7 PM. Essentially, you are skipping breakfast and lunch the following day during this method. Usually, someone following this method has one set day a week that they choose to follow this Intermittent fasting plan. It is best to review your schedule and find a day during the week that it will work best for you on a regular basis. For example, if you know that you are usually very busy on Monday and find it hard sometimes to sneak away for lunch already, maybe it would be an easy day to choose as your fasting day. On the other hand, if Friday is typically a day you like to rest and wrap up the week, it could be a great day to insert fasting into, setting you up for a nice Friday night meal as a reward for a week and fasting day well done.

It is not necessary to fast for a full 24 hours when following this method. Like the alternatives suggested in the 16/8 method above, you can choose to change the number of hours you want to fast. For example, for someone just starting with intermittent fasting and a history of "cheating" on diets, maybe a fasting period of 18 or 20 hours is best to start with. For those that have seen success with a shortened period or have a history of commitment to a plan, starting at 22 hours is a great place to begin. From there, you can work into a 24-hour fasting period. Additionally, you can start with one fasting period in a week and increase it to two if you feel inclined to. The following guide illustrates what it would look like to have a single day of fasting during the week at various times:

Week 1: Finish the last meal at 8 PM on Tuesday night, then do not eat again until 8 PM on Wednesday night.

Week 2: Finish the last meal at 8 AM on Monday morning, then do not eat again until 8 AM on Tuesday morning.

Again, you can play around with the times of this method to work for you. For example, instead of finishing eating at 8 AM, maybe you finish at 11 AM and do not eat again until 11 AM the next day. Find what times work best for you. If you are looking to shorten the time frame to 20 hours, you would finish a meal at 8 PM and begin eating again at 4 PM the following day. Use this as a starting point to adjust accordingly to your lifestyle and needs.

If "skipping" meals or cutting out food all together does not seem to fit with your goals or disposition, a third intermittent fasting method to consider is the 5/2 method. This refers to a period of five days during the week where you severely cut back on calories but eat normally the remaining five days of the week. Most of the time, on fasting days, people do not consume more than 600 calories in 24 hours. This allows for some food intake, but it is chosen very carefully and eaten mindfully so as not to go over the calorie goal. Women can cut that caloric goal further to see better results, lowering it to 500 calories on a fasting day. Men should stay closer to the 600 range. Like the 24-hour fast, it is best to look at your typical week and choose two days that would be best to dedicate to your Intermittent fasting. Some people like to choose Monday because of its start to the workweek, while others like to place their days in the middle of the week—Tuesday and Thursday. Also, you can begin with selecting one day a week to fast and cut back on caloric intake, building up to two days after you see success if you want.

A fourth method for intermittent fasting is called "Alternate-Day Fasting." This means that for one day you fast, the next day you do not, and so on. For most people, the fasting day consists of small amounts of food, about 500 to 600 calories total, similar to the plan mentioned above in the 5/2 method. If you find success with this method, you can try to go a full 24 hours with no food, and then 24 hours with food, and so on. It can be extreme to fast fully that regularly, so make sure to approach this concept with caution. In addition, this method can be hard to sustain a long-term plan. Some people follow this as a jumpstart for a week or two and then settle into one of the other methods. You can also adjust to doing one day on and two days off or eat more or fewer calories during fasting days as you see fit. There are more options here to explore, but again, it can be a hard method to follow, especially if you are new to intermittent fasting.

A more sustainable method that is actually a combination of both a more Paleo approach with an intermittent fasting component is called the "Warrior" diet. This plan was introduced and promoted by Ori Hofmekler, a fitness expert. Hofmekler recommends eating a small amount of food during the day and then enjoying a large meal in the evening. Daytime foods should primarily be fresh vegetables and fruits. The evening "feast" can contain unprocessed meats with whole foods and vegetables. The more closely associated with the food's natural state, the better, even when feasting at night. Remember, to see success with this plan, the fruit and vegetables consumed during the day still need to be minimal, while the meal at the end can be larger and full of a variety of nutrients. Of course, should you choose to explore this option, you can begin by adjusting your intake to fresh foods during the day and a regular meal at night, working your way into the full expression of the plan. This can be a sustainable meal plan for many people and worth exploring if you do not want to remove foods altogether. It can also be an ideal method for intermittent fasting for those that have pre-existing health conditions, which require constant nutritional intake.

The next intermittent fasting plan to consider is called the "Spontaneous Skip". For some people, their schedule varies from day-to-day, and it can be hard to pre-plan what meals will be skipped and when. In addition, some people do not thrive with such a rigid eating structure. It can be hard mentally as well as physically to know that you are about to enter a no-eating period or are in the throes of one with several more hours to go. Instead of setting up strict guidelines around your intermittent fasting, enjoy the benefits of this dieting plan by just telling yourself that you will miss a meal intentionally a couple of times during the week. You can give yourself permission to skip a meal if you are not hungry when lunchtime rolls around or just after waking up. You can also reassure yourself that you do not need to eat often especially if there is nothing appetizing for you at the moment. If you find you are too busy to cook something or to sit down for a healthy meal, maybe this is a time to do a short fast until you can enjoy eating a good meal again. The body does not need to consume food every few hours to stay functioning. In fact, your body is biologically wired to survive stretches of time without food, meaning it prepares for this time, whether you do it or not. All that preparation just sits in your storage room in your body, waiting for a time to use it. If you never use it, it just keeps filling up spaces in anticipation. This is why you get fat "pockets" that never seem to go away, even with intense exercise. What you really need is to give the body its natural opportunity to use its stored resources for energy.

Allowing yourself to spontaneously fast when the mood and timing are best for you helps you enjoy the benefits of intermittent fasting without the strict guidelines of other methods. Just make sure you try to stay consistent from week to week, setting a goal to skip maybe one or two meals a week, so you can benefit the most from this method. Also, try to select healthier foods when you are eating your "normal" meals during the rest of the week. This will also help make sure you get the most out of your intermittent fasting process. This bit of advice is applicable to any method you choose to implement and will be explored in more detail later in the book.

There are many published research papers and popular media figures that have followed a version of one of these methods with great success. Many people can find a "groove" and enjoy a new eating pattern that supports their overall health and weight goals. It is also a wonderful way to help lose unnecessary and stubborn weight and keep it off. One method is not a fit for every person, and no one should start in one particular place for the best results. It is an eating method and process that can be adapted to fit your life and needs and can also be tweaked as you move forward. That being said, below are some suggestions on how to find a method that works for your life and tips on how to adjust it over time.

How to Find Your Personal Intermittent Fasting Method

When you begin to explore a new lifestyle and eating process, you need to take a good look at your life. First, begin by examining your general traits. Select what traits you embody below:

o Stick to commitments	o Likes variety and spontaneity
o Easily accepts change	o Likes routine and familiarity
o Enjoys a challenge	o Prefers the "status quo"
o Has no health concerns or weight issues	o Works with medical professionals to manage health problems or weight maintenance

Next, consider your year. For example, do you know that you will be traveling somewhere for a business or personal trip? What about your plans for the holidays? Select a time to start your intermittent fasting lifestyle when you can have a period of at least four weeks back-to-back with minimal "special" interruptions. This includes birthdays for family members or other special occasions. These events are easy to adapt to, but when you begin, it is best to try to avoid these extra temptations. Identify a month where you have the least amount of these events.

Now, take a look at your week. Consider the following questions:

Question	Your Answer
What are your "best" days during the week?	
What is the "worst" day of the week for you?	
Do you tend to be a morning person or a night person?	
Do you like to go out to happy hour on Fridays or go out to parties on the weekend?	
What days of the week and times of day do you tend to have the most commitments?	
What time do you leave for work in the morning or get home in the afternoon or evening?	
What are your evening habits like?	

There are no "wrong" answers to these questions. Your responses should now be used to help you identify the best method for intermittent fasting for your life as it is now. As you being the process, you may notice some of your answers begin to change! That can be a great thing! Now, use the information above to determine the best method for you to follow and then outline how it will fit into your week. For example, if you know that you need to start off easy, like structure, and want to improve health and weight management, you will want to look at the methods that offer those benefits. From there, you can decide what month to begin, such as August, when there are no major holidays and you (theoretically) have no birthdays or travel plans scheduled. Then, using this information, you can identify the days of the week that you feel will be best for your fasting plans. Below are some of the pro's and con's for choosing a specific day to fast on:

Day of the Week	Pro	Con
Sunday	Great, empowering start	Last weekend day to feel freedom

	to the week	from commitment; church meal rituals for religious practitioners
Monday	Powerful control over a traditionally "hard" day of the week	Removing food as comfort on typically "stressful" days can be more harmful than helpful
Tuesday	A quiet day without much excitement allows for fewer distractions	Many meetings and activities occur in the evening on this day, making it hard to stay away from well-intentioned shared snacks or meal needs on the run

Wednesday	Similar to Monday, this day can be a "hard" day for people to deal with because it is the middle day and fasting can instill a sense of empowerment and control	Also like Monday, adding a stressor to an already "stressful" day can exacerbate the feelings rather than overcome them
Thursday	This day begins the wind-down of the work week and often comes with a lighter air than the start of the week, meaning a better mental attitude for fasting	As the "mood" becomes lighter, the desire for "celebratory" foods and activities are more common, such as early-week happy hours or get-togethers, making fasting more challenging
Friday	An excellent way	Many cultures

	to close a work week on your terms.	encourage after-work gatherings or lunchtime meals on this day, adding increased temptations
Saturday	The last day of the week can carry a great significance for faster's helping boost the sense of closing on a "good" note and securing another "win" before the weekends	This is often the first day free from work commitments, offering more free time to indulge; also, a religious day for some people, which also can come with rituals that involve food on this day

There is no "right" or "wrong" day or time to choose to fast. You will need to select the day that feels the best place to start for you. If you can only identify one day during the week that is more ideal for you than the others, then it is a great day to start on. If you can identify a few days during the week that you think could work, you have a variety of days to try out as you get started. Once you narrow down to the days during the week, you can narrow further to determine the times during the day. This also ties back into the type of intermittent fasting you have chosen to follow, but now is the time to look at your waking and sleeping habits, as well as your common mealtime habits. Once you determine this, you are set to begin your intermittent fasting process!

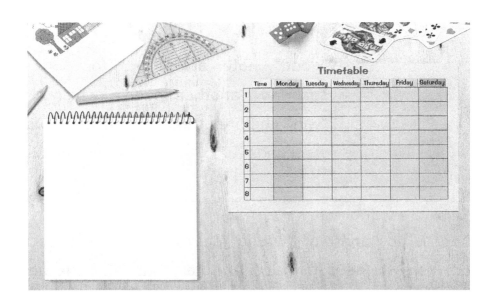

Chapter 4: Secret Techniques for Feasting on Your Favorite Foods

So, you may be thinking by this point, "Wait, I go hours, even days, without food?" Well, sort of. Maybe. When you are in a fasting period, you will have spans of time when you will decide if you want to consume nothing but non-caloric beverages, such as coffee, tea, and water, or if you want to stick to a plan that has minor or no caloric intake from foods. The reason for this is to prevent the body's insulin response from being active. You want the body to need to pull from the fat storage in your body for energy and fuel, not burn up what you are putting into it.

When you are breaking your fast and have a period of freedom in what and when you can eat, keep in mind that you need to ease in slowly. It is not the best idea to load up on carbs in your first meal after a fasting period. Doing this would send your insulin response system into "overdrive" right after a dormant period. Instead, try reaching for vegetables and fresh fruits. If you desire carbs, try a small serving of whole-grain pasta. Stay away from slices of bread and heavy carbohydrates for the first meal after a fast. This advice is contrary to people who are intensifying their workout during a fasting period. If this is the case for you, then a carb-heavy meal is necessary and your body will use those incoming fuel sources fast. It is also ill-advised to eat a very spicy meal right after fasting. This can cause indigestion and inflammation.

But these suggestions are just that: suggestions. If you have an iron stomach and are fine with spicy foods, then by all means, enjoy a good "hot" meal after your fast. You can still enjoy all your favorite foods while intermittent fasting, just mindfully on the days when you break your fast. The reason "mindfully" is mentioned here is because you not only want to watch what you reintroduce right after a fasting period, but you also want to keep an eye on your daily caloric intake. Remember, if you are looking to lose weight, your calories cannot be greater than your calories out. This means if you overeat on non-fasting days, also called "feasting" days, you will negate the progress you made during the fast. Instead, choose the foods you want to enjoy in relation to that calorie goal for the rest of the day.

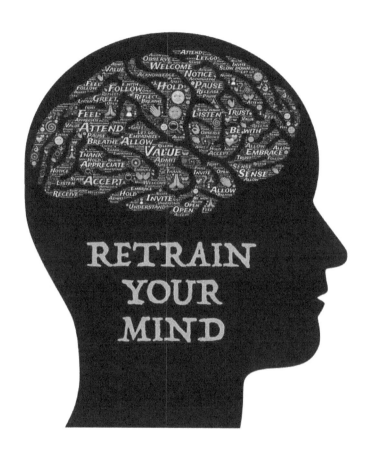

Another common question or concern is how often a person can eat during a "feasting" day. This is dependent on your preferences and your intermittent fasting plan. If you only have 8 hours to eat in, you can choose to eat all your calories in two large meals or three small meals, or just in snacking on healthy foods throughout the day. If you are doing a 24-hour fast and will not have another meal until dinnertime, you may eat a large dinner with a small snack later in the evening, but not much else during that day. You do not need to adhere to a "standard" meal plan with breakfast, lunch, and dinner occurring at specific times of the day. Instead, consider what times of the day you have to dedicate to eating well and what you prefer to do. Some people like the "visual" of "skipping" breakfast for his or her fasting, meaning they will not eat breakfast foods that day, but instead will eat a good lunch and dinner. Others will only count the hours of the fast and eat breakfast when the fast is broken, then adjust their meal times from there.

A word of caution for those considering the snacking option: be prepared with what you will "snack" on during your fasting days. Pre-packaged snacks tend to be heavy with carbs and calories, having little nutritional benefit. Preparing healthy meals are often more beneficial to your overall goals, but it requires more time on a feast day. If you want to snack throughout your day, plan ahead with healthy grab-and-go options you know will satisfy your hunger, calorie goals, and nutritional needs.

Always keep in mind that breaking your fast early or re-adjusting your needs throughout the process is acceptable and encouraged. This is supposed to be a sustainable meal planning process that fits into your life. If you feel, at hour 22, that you need to eat now or you will end up with a 48-hour fast because of your schedule, then eat! In addition, if you are in your first two weeks of adopting an intermittent fasting plan, and you find that one day is plenty and you do not want to do a full second day this week, take the day off or cut the fast shorter. Keep in mind, though, that the body requires about 13 hours for it to clear out remaining glucose and begin burning body fat. If you break your fast before 13 hours, you could be preventing your body from tapping into that backup energy storeroom. If you can, try to make it to 14 hours, if possible, but again, adjust as needed for your life. Another mental game you can play with yourself during this process is to see if you can extend the fasting period safely. For example, if you are doing a 16/8, what if you fasted for 17, giving yourself a window of 7 hours to eat your calories for the day? Trying to think about extending, rather than shortening, can make the time commitment not feel as stressed.

If you are starting off this process slowly and are cutting back on calories, stay within your selected calorie intake for the "fasting" day and then release the pressure of counting calories on the "feasting" day. Yes, it may take you longer to see results because you may be eating over your recommended calorie limit for your age and weight, but the idea is to give you the habit of fasting and then feasting. From there, you can begin to cut out food altogether during a fasting day or can begin counting calories on feasting days. It is up to you how you want to advance your intermittent fasting, so do not feel boxed into counting and restricting. Start with developing the habit first, and then move in the direction that makes the most sense for you.

Consider your favorite foods now. What are the foods that you love to go for when you treat yourself or want to indulge? These are foods you can still enjoy and savor when following an intermittent fasting plan. The caveat is that now you enjoy them on your feasting days or time window. If you are trying to lose weight and want results faster, take a look at the number of calories in these treats. How many treats can you eat within your feasting day or time frame without going over the calorie limit? For example, most women should stay below a 1,800 calorie day. If you know that your favorite ice cream has

500 calories per serving, you could only eat 3 servings of that ice cream, leaving 300 calories for other foods (hopefully with a nutritional content!). You may not want to dedicate all those calories on your feasting day to that ice cream, but what if you only had one scoop? What could you spend the rest of the 1,300 calories on? It could even be feasible to consider a half scoop of the ice cream, leaving you even more calories to allocate to other foods during the feasting time. If you love hamburgers, look at how many calories it contains and decide if you want the full burger or half of it. The same goes with a side of fries. Do you really need to eat the large portion or will you be happy with the small size and leaving more calories for something else later?

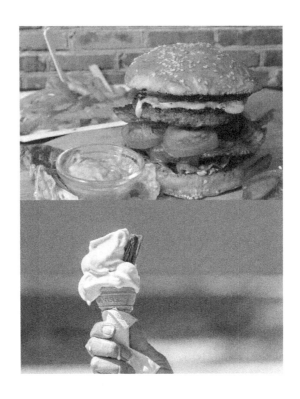

The wonderful thing about intermittent fasting is that you do not need to remove your favorite indulgences from your life forever. You are just selecting a specific time you will eat them, and if you want to go further with it, you will decide how much of it you want to eat during that time. You get to choose your own goals, time frame, and rules. As long as you are patient with the process, you can go as slow into the intermittent fasting plan as you want to. Remember in Chapter 1 about just cutting out a specific food for a day or two? This is a great example of starting in slowly, but your expectations need to match the speed. A slow start means a slow result. There is nothing wrong with that, in fact, it is a great place to be, but remember that as you measure your waist or step on the scale in the morning after a "fast" day. For those looking to lose weight more quickly, consider a more structured and restrictive approach while still falling within the appropriate guidelines. An alternate-day intermittent fast for two weeks with a healthy calorie limit on "feast" days can help you jumpstart your body's fat-burning process, but it requires a focused and committed approach. You may also not be able to enjoy many of your favorite foods during this two-week time frame. It is a tradeoff for speed, but it does not mean you have to say goodbye to chips, chocolate, or your other favorite foods for a long time and definitely not forever!

Below is a list of some of the more common "favorite foods" and their common calorie range. You can use this as a foundation for planning purposes. Explore what your favorite brands or foods are on your own to create your personal, customized favorite foods list to be more exact. You can follow the same format and design a list to reference when you need and want to. Keep in mind, this is a helpful tool for those that are restricting calories to a healthy range on the days that food is consumed or "feasting" days. This is not relevant to you if you are only focusing on caloric intake on fasting days. It is also not relevant for you if you do not want it to be! Choose to follow this or not, consume as much of your favorite foods on a feasting day as you want or find a limit. It is your call. And again, you can always start off slow, and then move into this phase of intermittent fasting.

Favorite Food and Drink	Common Calorie Range
Bagel	289
Beer, regular	153
Chocolate chip cookie	59
Soda, one cup	136
Graham cracker	59
Vanilla ice cream	145
Burger patty, no bun or toppings	193
Hot dog, no bun or toppings	137
Jelly donut	289
Ketchup, 1 tablespoon	15
Oatmeal, plain	147

Peanut butter, 2 tablespoons	180
Pepperoni pizza, one slice	298
Baked potato, no toppings	161
Salted potato chips, 1 ounce	155
Salted hard pretzels, 1 ounce	108
Ranch dressing, 2 tablespoons	146
Red wine, 5 ounces	123
White rice, 1 cup	205
Salsa, 4 ounces	35
Plain spaghetti, 4 ounces	221
Spaghetti sauce, 1 cup	92
White wine, 5 ounces	121
Chocolate-frosted vanilla cake, 1 piece	243
Bacon, 2 pieces	250
Sausage, pork, 2 pieces	250-290
Cream cheese	200
Chewing gum, 1 piece	9
Chocolate	200
Popcorn	150

White sugar, 1 teaspoon	20
Chik-Fil-A Waffle Fry, medium	360
Chik-Fil-A chicken sandwich	440
McDonald's french fries, medium	340
McDonald's hamburger	250
McDonald's chicken nuggets, 4 count	270
Taco Bell cheesy gordita crunch with shredded beef	500
Taco Bell nachos	310
Wendy's natural cut fries	228
Wendy's homestyle chicken sandwich	520
Wendy's Junior cheeseburger	280
Bread, white, 1 slice	96
Fried fish fingers or fish sticks, 1 piece	50
Lunch meats	300
Canned tuna, in water	100
Apple, 1	44

Banana, 1	107
Baked beans	170
Carrots	16
Celery	5
Dates	100
Olives	50
Orange	40
Peach	35
Pear	45
Pineapple	40
Plum	30
Strawberry, 1 large	10
Corn on the cob	70
Tomato	30
Cheese slice, 1 ounce	110
Cottage cheese	49
Egg, 1	90
Whole milk, 1 cup	175
Omelet with cheese	300
Plain yogurt	90
Butter, 1 tablespoon	112
Honey, 1 tablespoon	42
Jelly, 1 tablespoon	38

| Margarine, 1 tablespoon | 50 |
| Avocado | 150 |

Chapter 5: Tips and Tricks for Staying Motivated While Intermittent Fasting

It is not surprising to consider that "good" things will happen when you remove something "bad" from your diet. Meat is not really a "bad" thing, but fatty or meats that are harder to digest, such as red meat, can hurt the body, particularly if you eat a lot of it on a regular basis. This is why some people choose to remove some or all animal meat from their diet. In the case of someone doing an intermittent fast, this could mean cutting out meat for just the fasting portion of the diet plan. This is just one example of removing something "bad" for a time frame. Other "bad" foods to consider removing during an intermittent fasting regimen is fast food, processed foods, soda, and sugar.

Some of the "wins" for intermittent fasting occur in the small victories each day and week. For example, some people like to choose Friday as their fasting day because it ends the workweek. It gives people a "win" because they may have made "bad" choices all week, but on Friday, they get to end the week on a good note and start their weekend with a positive mindset. Other people like to start the week on Sunday or Monday with a fast, feeling like it provides a "fresh start" to the week. It sets them up for success for the rest of the week and is a positive "win" from the get-go. These are just a few tips for getting started in intermittent fasting.

Another suggestion for success includes approaching caloric restriction during intermittent fasting. You can choose what days and times are best to cut back on calories. Sometimes, you can cut back just a little bit during a small window of time, like cutting down to 1,300 calories for 6 hours, and then build from there, moving into 12 hours with a caloric intake no more than 500. After success here, maybe you move to a 24-hour fasting time frame. This can occur once a week to start, and then you can add more days as well if it fits with your schedule and lifestyle.

Part of the success of this method is more mental than physical. For example, when you choose to cut back on calories, you can pick a number that you think works, but for the best psychological success, cut your calories down by 25% to start. This is the average reduction that will show results. For a standard diet of 1,800 calories, for example, this means you would cut back to 1,350 for the fasting window. A great way to start this is simply to look at the calories overall and cut them back to this level. Once you master this after a few weeks, look into the types of calories you are consuming. Aim to select and remove foods that will accelerate your goals, such as removing carb-heavy foods. As you become more aware of the nutrition in the food you are consuming compared to the carb load it carries, you can begin to speed up the results of your efforts. Easing into this level of awareness is often beneficial so you do not feel overwhelmed and confused. First, start with just reducing calories by a certain percentage, and then maybe bringing more awareness to your food, or maybe increasing the percentage further, such as up to 45%.

Another tip for introducing intermittent fasting into your life is by timing it to occur overnight while you are sleeping. For example, instead of fasting during the day and then cramming in calories right before bed, plan your fasting hours around your typical meal times. For example, if you normally wake up about 6:30 AM, eat breakfast about 7 AM, lunch about 11 AM, and dinner from 7:30 PM to 8 PM, you have a great place to start from. Consider not eating anything after 8 PM when you finish your dinner and then adjust your breakfast time to 8 AM. This means you are only pushing your mealtime by an hour! If that is tough, what if you ate dinner a half hour earlier, at 7 PM, resulting in your finishing at 7:30 PM? Then, do not eat breakfast the following morning until 7:30 AM. This way you are only adjusting 30 minutes on each end. That is feasible, right?

While this plan may sound okay on paper, it can pose a challenge for many. For example, do you like to "snack" after dinner? Are you prone to grabbing a bag of chips while you watch your favorite show until bedtime? Do you make yourself a cocktail when you clean up in the evening? Are you known for grabbing a bowl of ice cream or a piece of chocolate after you put the kids to bed? Choosing to conduct your intermittent fasting overnight means nothing but water and (most likely) decaffeinated coffee or tea after dinner is over. If you find it a challenge to stay away from the snacks and "midnight" treats, consider trying to get to bed earlier on during these fasting nights. Take a look at your typical routine and find a balance that will work best for you. You can even try out a few combinations to find what is most comfortable with your life and schedule.

For those of you that are looking to take fasting to the next level and are considering implementing an alternate-day fasting plan, make sure to start off the process slow. To begin, try fasting for a period of 6 hours during the day. After success with this for a couple of weeks, increase fasting to 8 hours, then 12, and aim for 24 hours in the end. It is okay for those following this plan to consume whatever you want on a "feast" day or during non-fasting hours. Sometimes, it can be a nice reprieve to not have to worry about caloric intake after restricting food for an entire day. Also, make sure to drink plenty of fluids during your fast. Just make sure those drinks do not have any added calories in the form of sweeteners, flavorings, or cream. Coffee, tea, still water, and sparkling water are all good options to have on hand at all times during the fasting period.

If an alternate fasting schedule seems like a challenge, consider setting your fasting hours to 6 or 8 hours during the fasting day and instead of cutting out food altogether, begin with reducing your calories to a fraction of what you normally intake. For example, start by cutting back by 25%, then move to 50%, and then 75%, leading up to 100% of calories being restricted. Cutting back calories for these times is a more gentle way for implementing the alternate-day intermittent fasting process that can still show great results. To also help with this plan, aim to ingest the majority of calories in the evening in the form of a large, well-rounded dinner.

Some people are concerned about their nutritional intake during and after fasting. If you are making sure you eat well-rounded and healthy meals during your non-fasting days, you will be able to get all the nutrition you need. But if you are not watching what you eat on the "off" days (or "on" depending on how you look at it!), vitamins are a nutritional source to consider. In the beginning, you may have trouble just getting a handle on the intermittent fasting process and not even dig into the nutrition of the food you consume on your fasting days. That is fine! This means, however, that your nutrients may be a little off. Taking a good multi-vitamin or a mix of various vitamins to make sure you are getting what you need is a good place to start. If you have never taken a combination of vitamins before, know that taking these on an empty stomach can be a little upsetting. Make sure you have some food in there before taking them, if possible. For fasting days, when you are not eating and have no food in your stomach, liquid forms of the vitamins are easier on your digestion, therefore making it more pleasant to your tummy. If that still bothers you, consider spacing out the vitamins throughout the day so it is not so much at one time. These small doses, even taken frequently daily, are a great way to also fuel your body with nutrients it needs but without the calories.

In addition, you can look for vitamins that offer an additive that makes you feel full or helps suppress your appetite. On a fasting day, this can be comforting, especially when you are feeling the throes of hunger coming on. Try taking a vitamin like this in the middle of the day when you would normally have lunch or an afternoon snack. Also, vitamins that tend to hurt your stomach can be taken right before you go to bed. The discomfort is less obvious when you are resting. It is a natural mechanism your body does for you that you can take advantage of. Remember to be consistent with your vitamins and the time of day you take them. When you implement intermittent fasting into your life your body has to learn to adjust to a whole new way of fueling itself. The more continuity you can offer it, such as vitamins entering your body at a certain time every day, the better it will cope with the changes.

As mentioned earlier, a multi-vitamin that offers 100% of your daily nutritional needs and is also calorie-free is an excellent option to consider. That being said, these pills are often large and can punch the gut hard when they hit, especially on a fasting day when there is no food in the stomach to soften it. If you have trouble handling a single multi-vitamin, try breaking it up to take throughout the day, as mentioned earlier, or come up with your own concoction of essential vitamins that you can spread out separately so it is easier on the tummy. To help you identify the top important vitamins and the doses for a typical healthy adult, the following list is a guide to start from. You can also use this guide to help find a multi-vitamin if you are looking for a single pill to take.

Vitamin	Dose	Notes
Vitamin A	5,000 IU	Look for Retinol
Vitamin B1	1.5 mg	

Vitamin B2	1.7 mg	
Vitamin B3	20 mg	
Vitamin B5	10 mg	
Vitamin B6	2 mg	
Vitamin B7	300 micrograms	
Vitamin B9	400 micrograms	
Vitamin B12	6 micrograms	
Vitamin C	60 mg	You cannot overdose on this, so the more the merrier if you like
Vitamin D	400 IU	Look for D3
Vitamin E	30 IU	
Vitamin K	80 micrograms	
Choline	400 mg	For a healthy liver, muscle, and nerve function
BCAA's, or Branch Chain Amino Acids	Check the bottle for dosing recommendations	Helps promote the feeling of being full and supports the

		muscles from breaking down

You can control the time of year when you fast for the best results. Intermittent fasting is more of an eating plan and lifestyle than a fad diet. This means you need to approach it with the understanding that this is something you will embrace for a long time. So, when is the best time of year to start this process? That is up to you and your upcoming few months or even year. Take a look at your calendar and see what you already have planned for the future. No, there is never a "perfect" time to start this. There will always be something that can tempt you to fall off your path for well-being but look for a time when you have a couple of weeks with nothing major planned. Do you have a big conference coming up in July, and you know that you will only have a bagged meal to snag on your way to the next presentation? That is not a good time to start. Do you know that your best friend is getting married in October or a big celebration is going to happen in March? Those are times to encounter when you are already an intermittent fasting professional (or at least have a few wins under your belt), not when you are first starting out. Any big event or major routine change can knock you off balance with your intermittent fasting goals. Instead, look at those weeks when you have a "normal" routine. The success of a win, such as every time you make it through another fasting period, is vital. When you tempt yourself or put yourself in a situation that this can be extra-hard, you deprive yourself of the opportunity for this win. Consider implementing your intermittent lifestyle before a big event if you have at least 4 weeks prior to stock up a few wins and establish a good routine. If you do not have this time, maybe wait until after to start it up. Having a setback, especially right in the beginning, can be a blow that is hard to recover from. Choose your starting date wisely.

Also, mentioned earlier in this book, the days of the week you choose for fasting should also be chosen with care. If you turn back to the breakdown of the pro's and con's for each day of the week, you can begin to formulate what days you should consider for your fasting days and for your feasting days. For example, if you want to start your week off on a "clean slate" and on the "right foot", fasting can be a great way to get ready for the week ahead. On the other hand, if you always celebrate the start of the week with a mini-mourning session filled with cocktails and chocolate, choosing Sunday or Monday for a fasting day may end up being torture instead of positive. Instead, consider fasting on Tuesday and Thursday. Also, some people live for the weekend and the indulgences of boozy brunches, happy hours, small plates, and late-night munchies. Choosing to fast on Friday or Saturday could be a horrible plan and do nothing but set them up for failure. These people may do better with fasting days on Monday and Wednesday. This leaves Sunday for a recovery day and ends right before the weekend begins to kick up. If a person is looking to expand their fasting to 3 days and still wants to keep the weekends open, Thursday is still available as an additional day.

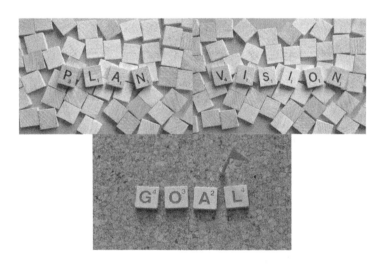

You can always move around the days you choose to fast on, but try to choose a day or two and stick with it for at least two weeks. After two weeks, adjust to better suit your needs. The same goes for picking the hours of the days you want to fast. This was introduced earlier but bears repeating because of its importance to your success with intermittent fasting. You need to choose times during the day that make the most sense for you. Earlier the concept of fasting overnight was suggested, but that may not work well for you if you are doing a 24-hour fast and always eat breakfast. People that love a good, hearty breakfast should consider fueling up in the morning and then starting their fast at 7 AM, then not eating again until breakfast time the following morning where they can eat another good breakfast before the day starts. Following a plan like this allows the body to burn off the food consumed in the morning throughout the day anyway because your body is more active, therefore, the metabolism also is more active. If you are not doing a 24-hour fast, play around with the hours you would choose to fast to make sure you set yourself up for success. For example, consider the person who loathes Mondays and always mourns the day with a bog cocktail at 6 PM and a good sweet treat. If they are starting their fast on

Monday morning at 9 AM, then they would not be eating again until 9 PM, if they are doing a 12-hour fast. This is just bad news for this person! It is unnecessary pain and suffering! Instead, they should consider starting their fast at 6 PM on Sunday night so they can wake up Monday and have a good breakfast at 6 AM and the rest of the day to indulge as desired. Maybe one day, a fast or change to their habits will be something to consider, but when you are first starting out to stay motivated, choose times that will support you.

Increasing intensity is possible and encouraged. Start off by "dipping your toes" into intermittent fasting by using the method that suits you best. Start off small and slow, giving yourself at least 2 weeks to adjust to the changes.

Then, decide how you want to increase and when. For example, some people may start with reducing caloric intake on one day a week. After a few weeks of success, they may decide to increase the caloric restriction until they finally reach the end goal of complete fasting for 12 or 24 hours. Another person starting intermittent fasting at the same time may decide to instead increase the time frame of their fasting from 12 hours to 18, and then ultimately to 24. Or another may decide to add a second fasting day to their week. Decide on a goal that you want to achieve and start working there bit by bit, week by week. Once you achieve that goal and can maintain it for 4 weeks, determine a new goal and start working towards that one.

Maybe your ultimate goal is 24-hour fast several days during the week! Just keep working up the intensity after you hit a goal and allow your body time to adjust and balance.

It will always take a little time to get comfortable with a new routine. Sometimes, it is nice to find something working and keep with that for weeks on end before you introduce a new change. That is good, too! This plan is not about a quick fix or a "crash" diet. This is about a long-term healthy eating plan that maintains your weight and wellbeing.

Give yourself the time to settle into that.

Chapter 6: How Fasting Works to Safely Increase Weight Loss

The secret is out, ladies! The "newest" diet trend that is sweeping the nation is intermittent fasting. It is helping people shed an impressive number of pounds and keep them off while adding a whole lot of other benefits to their lives. But here is something fascinating you may know by now: this "miracle" weight loss plan is nothing new, and it is not the "crash" diet that some people are making it out to be. It is a popular lifestyle that many people have used with great success for thousands of years. Like other popular nutritional plans today, it's about looking back to pave the way for the future. Nutritionists, dieticians, fitness experts, doctors, and scientists alike are beginning to embrace what has been used for centuries to do everything from curing a cold to stopping heart problems, as well as lose weight healthily. This mentality can also explain why many people who choose to follow the Paleo or the "caveman's" diet, are also big supporters of intermittent fasting, both mimic the eating habits of ancient ancestors. Our brains have not caught up to our current evolution, meaning that they are still operating like cavemen. Therefore, it makes sense to mimic this natural eating pattern for the best results in our bodies.

You may hear some people call intermittent fasting a weight loss "hack" or a "magic pill" for keeping off the unwanted pounds, but you should be able to recognize by now the powerful benefits of this ancient technique. But to better understand how it helps you lose and keep off weight, you need to dig into the science a bit more. First, you must understand the biological reaction that occurs when the body runs out of glucose. When you eat food, the body changes it into various nutrients to use in the body. One of those is sugar, which is then released into the bloodstream as glucose. This is what the body will use first for energy. This is why you get a spurt of energy when you eat something with a lot of sugar but crash hard when it wears off. This is your body reacting to the increase in energy but then diving down when it is used up. When your body runs out of the glucose coursing through your blood, it needs to turn somewhere else to gather its energy from. This is when it turns to your fatty deposits.

Any time you consume calories and nutrients that are not used up in the energy-burning process, your body tucks away that energy for a "rainy" day. In cavemen days, this meant that the extra calories consumed on one day got stored in their body to cover them until they got to eat again, which was sometimes several days later. Your body is still thinking it is a caveman without constant access to nutrients. Your body has been preparing for the day when you do not have something to eat. When your glucose is gone, you are giving your body that moment it has been preparing for! Now, it can tap into that stored fat to retrieve your needed energy. Now, you are burning calories very differently. You are not just losing bloating from too much salt or dropping "water weight", but you are depleting your stubborn fat pockets that seem to never go away no matter how many squats or sit-ups you do. This is why you lose weight and inches around the body. It is also why your skin will glow and you will look healthy. You are using a natural, biological process to lower to a healthy weight and maintain it.

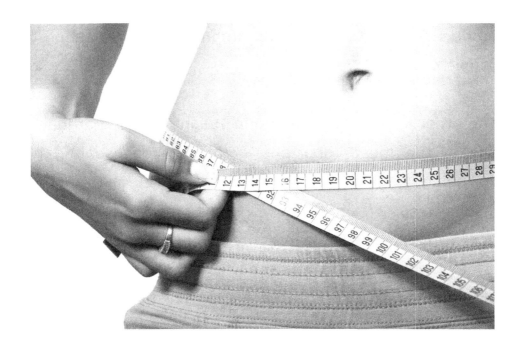

Another added weight-loss benefit is the release of hormones in the body that aid in burning off fat. The first hormone to consider is HGH, or the Human Growth Hormone. It is what fires up your fat burning process when glucose is out of the picture so your body can gather the energy required for daily functioning. In some published studies, it was found that women's HGH production increased by up to 1,300% while fasting! Athletes have been using or avoiding synthetic HGH for years to improve their overall athletic abilities, but maybe they did not know that they can naturally increase their production by a substantial amount just by fasting a couple of days a week!

The other important hormone in weight loss and arguably one of the most important factors in your health and wellbeing is insulin. Maintaining a stable, low level of insulin keeps off and removes extra fat. You gain weight and raise your insulin levels when you eat foods that have a lot of simple sugar, like soda, cookies, and candy, and also with a lot of processed carbs, like rice, pasta, and bread. Every time you eat something in those categories, your insulin levels jump up and then dive back down. It is the opposite of being low and stable. When this happens, your body is programmed to stock away from the extra fats and sugars you are taking in for "emergencies" or later on down the road when food is scarce. The problem is that, for most people, food is not scarce and there are no "sustenance emergencies". Therefore, the more you eat of these foods, the more your body stores away. Every time you jump up your insulin levels, you bring yourself closer and closer to a dangerous disease—type 2 diabetes. You also inch yourself closer to obesity if you are not there already. Elevated insulin levels can also lead to many more chronic illnesses, so it needs to be avoided at all costs. Amazingly, intermittent fasting is a great solution to this problem. In clinical studies, participants that followed an intermittent fasting regimen for a little over 2 weeks showed a natural "balance" in their insulin levels. This occurred for not only those that were pre-diabetic or showing a disposition for developing type 2 diabetes in the future, but also for people already suffering from diabetes. Insulin injections are known to be hard on the liver and kidneys as well as other internal organs but naturally balancing the hormone level is a safe and clinically proven successful method for finding it. This balanced state is what allows your body to continue to burn fuel rather than store it. It is also a great energy booster throughout the day, which is an added perk of this health and weight loss plan.

Another benefit of intermittent fasting and weight loss is the impact on your hunger hormones. Hunger is a two-part process. One part is physical; when your stomach is empty, it sends a message to the brain that you need food. This is a biological response. The other process is chemical, which is triggered when the body anticipates when it is about to eat. Think about when it gets close to your "normal" lunchtime. You begin to feel hungry, even if you just ate something fulfilling a few minutes ago. This is because you have trained your chemical response to anticipating food coming around this time, and therefore, the message was sent to the brain to prepare for it. During intermittent fasting, you begin to break these chemical habits. You no longer have "normal" time for eating food because you have changed it up on the body. You will have these urges for a few days, maybe even up to a couple weeks, but you will be able to "retrain" these chemicals to anticipated a new eating schedule. This means those hunger pangs and cravings will diminish or even be eliminated. When you have fewer tugs on your tummy from these pains and cravings you have better success sticking to your diet plan and seeing more success as a result.

There is a myriad of factors that influence the amount of weight you will lose. Some of those factors include what foods you consume on "feasting" days, the length and frequency of your fasts, and the consistency of your fasting schedule. Every week, you can lose up to 3 pounds of stored fat if you consistently fast for about 15 hours per day. And the nice part is that you really do not need to "count calories" or cut out your favorite foods to make this happen! A study published in 2018 showed that overweight adults lost an average of 15 pounds between 3 and 12 months. Another published study revealed that overweight adult participants lost up to 8% of their body weight in as little as 3 weeks and up to 24. In addition, the study published that the participant's waist circumference shrunk by up to 7% in the same time frame! Imagine losing 8% of your body weight in 3 weeks! For an adult who weighs 250 pounds, this means a possible loss of 20 pounds in less than a month. That is pretty good!

Another thing that can impact the amount of weight you can lose is your exercise habits. You are able and encouraged to work out while intermittent fasting. You can do just about any form of exercise, and it will benefit your efforts, but there are some that will speed up your weight loss more than others. For example, if you do up to four high-intensity workouts during the week, partnered with consistent intermittent fasting, you can expect to shed pounds much faster than no or little activity with fasting. Work on bursts of activity during these exercise sessions, trying not to rest too much between each repetition or set. This approach will encourage additional caloric removal. This approach also helps build up your muscles, making your body look and feel healthy and strong.

A lot of people assume that the weight they will lose while intermittent fasting will be in the form of muscle mass. What is unique about this diet plan is that it hits a "sweet" spot for weight loss. You need to fast for much longer than 24 hours to lose muscle mass. Your body will not start breaking down muscles for energy until usually day 4. This means you could technically do a fast for 3 days and still be only burning stored fat before it even considers going to your muscles for energy. You need to give your body several hours to burn through the residual glucose in your bloodstream before it gets into your fat stores, typically about 14 hours, but once it gets in there, you are going to use up your fat before anything else. And the more fat you have stored, the more it will take from there before touching your lean muscle.

As mentioned in the previous chapter, you can also take nutritional supplements to help your body while fasting, especially if you are new at this. You want to make sure your nutritional needs are met, and taking a multi-vitamin or a few different key vitamins are a great way to do this until you figure out how to balance your food intake. If you are working out frequently and intensely during your fasting periods, consider taking the BCAA's to help stabilize your energy levels and provide additional support to your muscles.

All About Ketosis

When you fuel your body with fat, your body enters into a natural state of being called "ketosis". This almost always occurs when you fast or when you restrict carbohydrates on a regular basis, such as when following a Keto diet. The reason people want to enter ketosis is for its various benefits, including weight loss, improved overall health markers, and enhanced performance. Unfortunately, it can be a dangerous state for some people, such as type 1 diabetics. This is why you should know your body and work with a physician if you have a condition that can be impacted by a state of ketosis. Otherwise, there are ways to harness the power of this instinctual state of being without the negative side effects. To begin, it is important to know exactly what ketosis is.

Small little molecules lie in wait to fuel the body called "ketones". This is what the "keto-" in the word "ketosis" comes from. These molecules are developed from the consumed fat and become activated when glucose is low or non-existent. Low levels of protein and very minimal carbs in a diet can produce extra ketones in the body. Excessive amounts of protein are turned into blood sugar, which is why protein should be consumed at moderate levels. When there is not enough glucose to fuel the body, the fat is processed through the liver and is turned into ketones. These ketones move into the bloodstream like glucose would have to fuel your body. Their function is similar to glucose once it reaches your bloodstream. The brain even thrives off ketones instead of glucose. This is critical to the success and health of your body because the fat cannot fuel the brain directly and it requires an immense amount of fuel.

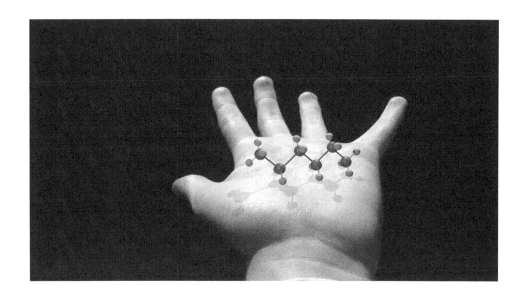

Each time you enter into a fasting period during your intermittent fasting process, the body switches from running on glucose and sugar to running on ketones and fat. When this happens, your insulin levels drop low and find a stable space so that the burning of your fat can increase. This is one of the easiest methods for getting at your fatty deposits in your body and getting rid of them once and for all! The benefits and results of approaching weight loss this way far exceed any other traditional diet plan, including Paleo. The fastest way for your body to enter ketosis, or a state of being where there are significant levels of ketones in the blood, is through fasting. A "significant level" means more than 0.5 mM of ketones in the bloodstream. However, once you break a fast, your body will lose the ketosis state, meaning you have to "start over" again the next time you fast. This is also a natural fluctuation for your body.

When your body enters ketosis, you offer your brain and body a practically unlimited amount of energy. Your body has fatter than it can burn through in several days, even months sometimes. When you find yourself in ketosis, the energy increases, the physical endurance improves, the mental clarity enhances, hunger pains reduce, and weight loss improves. It is also a natural treatment for type 2 diabetes and has been shown to permanently "heal" this illness is a variety of human trials. Another common disease treated with ketosis is epilepsy. Many people who follow a keto diet or use intermittent fasting can control their epilepsy for the long-term without medication! There are so many additional benefits beyond or associated with losing weight when entering into a state of ketosis.

To enter a state of ketosis faster each time you fast, you can observe a ketogenic diet on your "feasting" days. This is basically a very low-carb and low-protein diet plan. More on this diet method will be discussed later in the book. When you combine the two, you encourage your body to enter and hover around the state of ketosis, if not remaining in it for a long time.

You will know when you enter into a state of ketosis. You can measure it with breath, blood, or urine samples, though there are some other signs that do not require any testing. Some of the most common ways to tell you are in ketosis is the minimization of discomfort and hunger, as well as increased energy and mental clarity. If you want to make sure you are in a state of ketosis, you can consider purchasing special testing equipment such as a blood ketone meter, breath ketone analyzers, or urine strips that show ketone levels.

Sometimes, people experience negative side effects when they enter into a state of ketosis. For example, some study participants have complained of heart palpitations, constipation, cramping in the legs, increased agitation, lethargy, and headaches. Most of the time the side effects are temporary and minor disturbances. In addition, these are almost always tied to sodium and hydration levels. To prevent or remove these side effects, eat a little salt or drink a lot of water and give it a few minutes. Most likely in about 5 minutes, the negative feelings will be gone.

The biggest challenge to you is more about how to reach the optimal level of ketosis for weight loss and health. This is not a cut-and-dry process; there is a range of ketosis that people float back and forth in. You will start to see a difference when you get to 0.5 mM or millimolar. You will continue to see optimal results between 0.5 and 3.0. When you reach over 3.0 mM, you begin to move into "starvation" mode and are no longer in a healthy range. This means you need to eat a healthy meal with good carbs to bring your levels back down. If your levels reach about a 10 mM, you are entering into a state called "ketoacidosis". This can be a very dangerous state of being, which most often occurs to type 1 diabetes patients who do not control their insulin. It is a rare malfunction in the body, while ketosis is a natural and healthy state. These two are very different, but can sometimes be confused with one another.

Ketosis is a controlled state of being. Most people struggle to get to the 0.5 mM mark, let alone venture up to the 3.0 mM mark. In rare instances do people who are truly starving get beyond 7.0 mM. In a healthy body, it is almost impossible to enter into ketoacidosis. They may sound similar and have to do with similar ketones, but they are very distinct states of being. When a body is in ketoacidosis, their ketones are excessive in the bloodstream. This results in extreme pain in the stomach and nausea or vomiting, and then mental "fog" before coma and death. Medical treatment is required and is an urgent condition. This is very different from ketosis and not something you could easily enter into while on intermittent fasting without an underlying medical condition, such as type 1 diabetes. If you fear you are reaching a starvation level or even ketoacidosis, you can prevent this from worsening by simply eating a healthy number of carbs to reduce ketones and introduce glucose back in for a while.

Chapter 7: The Process of Autophagy and Why It Is So Important for Women

The activation and improved functioning of your body occur through autophagy. Don't worry if you have never heard of this before, many people not have. But it is well worth knowing about, especially for women. Learning about the process of autophagy and how you can use it to feel and look younger is not a trick, but more of an empowering art form.

When you participate in intermittent fasting, you begin to burn mostly fat for energy. This is what activates autophagy in your body. The process of autophagy is translated from the Greek word's "auto" and "phagy". The two terms together mean "self-eating". This may sound terrible on the surface, but when you begin to understand what it is referring to, you will see the benefit in this natural process. The idea of self-eating is actually applied at the cellular level. When your body enters into autophagy, the process begins consuming the unnecessary organelles, then reuses a part of the cells as building blocks for other body functions. It is a powerful and necessary process everyone has. The unfortunate problem is that things like toxins in your environment and a diet high in processed foods begin to reduce autophagy. Typically, this process takes place overnight as you rest your body. In addition, when you eat meals high in fat and use your fat to fuel your body, you are activating autophagy.

There are other ways to activate autophagy, including certain exercises and consuming caffeine. EGCGs in green teas are also known to stimulate the process of autophagy. One of the great benefits of these, in particular, is the activation in the skin, making it "glow" and be healthy.

You can clean and detox your cells with autophagy that you stimulate during intermittent fasting. Introducing clean proteins and healthy fats on your feast days is also an excellent way to encourage autophagy. Most people need to do this on a regular basis for the best results. This is what sets intermittent fasting apart from other similar diets, such as the Keto diet and Paleo diet. These two plans, in particular, encourage a high amount of protein or other sources of calories, which can prevent autophagy. Intermittent fasting provides the body to work with the fat stores as energy sources and also cleanse the body at the cellular level. Not many other dieting plans can say it can do that!

As you allow and encourage your body to work through the process of autophagy, you are giving the cells of your body the chance to clear out the gunk and toxins that have been building up. This heals your body on the cellular level and makes it shine "from the inside out", which means you are cleaning out the tarnish in your body that is keeping you from being healthy and full of energy and also what is keeping you from looking your best on the outside, such as glowing skin, healthy nails, and lustrous hair.

What many people still do not recognize is the medical advancement this process is exposing. In 2016, the biologist from Japan won a Nobel Prize for the study on autophagy and the human body. Thanks to this notoriety, more and more scientific studies have been conducted and published. It has been shown to positively impact those suffering from cancers and various neuro-degenerative illnesses. It has also been linked to helping prevent these diseases from manifesting. What is reassuring is that every cell in your body has the process of autophagy in it. You just need to give it a chance to do its job, and one of the best ways to do that is through intermittent fasting.

Think of autophagy in terms of making a meal in your kitchen. You cook the food, clean up afterward, throw out some food, and keep others for later. When you go back into your kitchen the next day, it is clean and ready to work again. This is like your cells and the process of autophagy. Your cell is the kitchen. It works hard, and then you start the process of "cleaning" it up afterwards or autophagy. You keep some things, toss others, and get it ready to work again.

Now, think about later in life, as you begin to age, and you are not as diligent about "cleaning" up after making a meal. This can happen because of lifestyle impact or from environmental exposure to various toxins. Whatever prevents the autophagy process to function properly or well means that a lot of junk gets left "on your kitchen counters". The longer it sits in your cells, the more toxic it becomes. It begins to smell, contaminate other things, and make the space unbearable for life. This is what can happen to your cells if you are not careful. This is why this process is so important to know, understand, and encourage.

From a biological standpoint, a woman's body is very different from a man's. When you recognize this and support the female body specifically, it can thrive and glow. This can include things like self-care and self-calming activities, like meditation. It also means consuming fluids, like water and coffee or tea to help jumpstart the metabolism and process of autophagy. This also means following an intermittent fasting process to support autophagy and all the other healthy process kick-started while fasting.

It is great to start the process of intermittent fasting and the support of autophagy by removing simple sugars from your diet. Then, from there, you should increase the amount of healthy fat you eat during a feasting day. For example, when you are about to break your fast, choose food with a lot of healthy fat. This could be olive oil, avocado, or another source of good fat. In fact, most of your diet should be fat-focused. But remember to also make sure the fat is "good". In addition, choose foods with a good amount of polyphenols. Once you reintroduce food into your diet and begin with fat, you can then mix in a few carbs and a good amount of fiber.

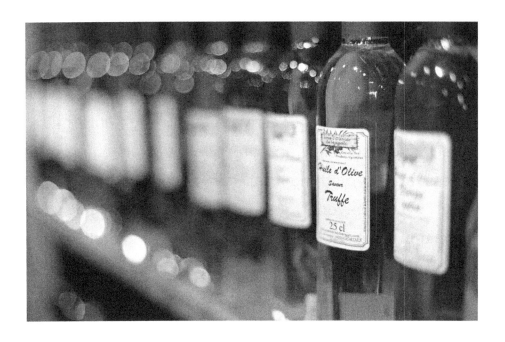

When you go back into fasting, the more fat you provided to your body during the "feasting" period, the more quickly your body will adapt to fueling with fat instead of glucose. In addition, the minimal introduction of glucose and sugar into your body during a feast day means that your body will not have much to burn through, getting to the fat faster and faster each time you fast. This speeds up the benefits of intermittent fasting, including health and weight loss goals.

Embracing this process can completely change your relationship and response to food. It forces you to approach eating in a different manner than what has been popularized in the media for years before. But the science cannot lie about the benefits of this process on your body and how to activate it through intermittent fasting, exercise, diet, and lifestyle. It is an empowering process and something that can transform your life in many ways beyond just health and weight. Your connection to foods and cravings can completely change as you embrace this process and the idea of healthy fat over calories and carbs.

One great way to improve your mental clarity and increase energy levels is by consuming an "autophatea". This is also known to help reduce the risk of heart disease and neurodegenerative diseases. It is also a good tea to drink during feast or fast mornings because it is a low- or no-calorie beverage. Consuming fat first thing in the morning can help you be fulfilled until you break your fast in the afternoon if that is your fasting schedule. It also helps reduce the hunger cravings and boosts your metabolism for the rest of the day.

You can also consider sipping on this beverage before a workout or an intense part of your day. The caffeine is a nice energy-booster and can also support fat burning while engaging in physical activity. You can have up to 4 cups of this tea per day for the best results. After 2 PM, consider changing to a decaffeinated version. Another good tip for this tea is to ensure the Earl Grey tea you purchase is whole citrus, not a synthetic version. This means it is lacking the high-quality ingredients necessary for activating your autophagy process.

How to Brew Your Tea

Ingredients:
1 bag, whole-citrus Earl Grey tea
1 bag, green tea (organic is best)
1 tbsp, coconut oil (raw)
1 stick, cinnamon (Ceylon is best)
1 tsp, powder of monk fruit (as preferred)

Instructions:
1. Boil between 1 and 1.5 cups of water and pour into a large teacup or mug.
2. Place the 2 tea bags and cinnamon stick into the cup. Set a timer to let the ingredients steep for at least 3 minutes. You can let it steep longer but the water will begin to cool. Remove the stick and bags.
3. Stir in the coconut oil, using the cinnamon stick, for about 30 seconds.
4. If you are incorporating it, stir in the powder of monk fruit with the cinnamon stick as well. Enjoy warm!

More on the Science of Autophagy and Women

Below is a sample of a few different scholarly and professional articles that discuss and support the role of autophagy in health, particularly for women. What follows is a citation for the article and a brief summary of the content of the study. If you are interested in reading more of the study, follow the links provided for access to the full text.

Study #1: On the Role of Autophagy in Human Diseases:

A Gender Perspective.

Link: https://www.ncbi.nlm.nih.gov/pmc/articles/PMC3823190/

Citation: "Lista, P., Straface, E., Brunelleschi, S., Franconi, F., & Malorni, W. (2011). On the role of autophagy in human diseases: a gender perspective. *Journal of cellular and molecular medicine*, *15*(7), 1443-57."

Several expected and unexpected impacts on disease and health by autophagy have proven to degrade systolic proteins in lysosomes. This means that the prevention of neurodegeneration and cancer is possible through autophagy because it adds to the adaptive and innate longevity and immunity of various important proteins in the body. For example, in the heart, under normal conditions, autophagy is necessary for the change in low-level basal organelles. When there is heart disease or other stress on the heart, like reperfusion or ischemia, the response is up-regulated. This shows that the death or survival of a cell is tied to autophagy's role in elucidation. Based on the results of this study, it can be hypothesized that several human diseases and conditions can be significantly impacted by the manipulation of autophagy. In addition, it is necessary to further study the role of autophagy and targeted drugs and pathogenic mechanisms. This is partly in response to the increased research in gender disparity in molecular and cellular performance in diseases such as heart disease, immune disease, cancer, and neurodegeneration. Gender-specific therapy in the future could also be impacted because there is a strong relationship between hormones and autophagy. There is also a strong connection between the process of autophagy and the sex of a cell. Note that men and women are predisposed and sensitive to different illnesses and respond differently to different, current treatment therapy. This is due to the physiological differences between men and women. This makes the study of gender variance and the process of autophagy pivotal in the process of developing more effective strategies for therapy.

Study #2: Sex Differences in Autophagy Contribute to Female Vulnerability in Alzheimer's Disease.

Link: https://www.ncbi.nlm.nih.gov/pmc/articles/PMC6023994/

Citation: "Congdon E. E. (2018). Sex Differences in Autophagy Contribute to Female Vulnerability in Alzheimer's Disease. *Frontiers in neuroscience*, 12, 372. doi:10.3389/fnins.2018.00372."

It is known in the Alzheimer's disease community that there is a difference between genders regarding the risk and development of the disease. It is also known that there are clear deficits in the process of autophagy for Alzheimer's patients. When examining the intersection of autophagy and the intersection with sex and disease, it is possible that the reduction in autophagy can increase the risk of development. Women are more prone to developing Alzheimer's disease than men. They are also more likely to have a more severe manifestation of the disease than men. This is the result of several aspects of the lifespan of the person. One of these aspects is the double-X chromosome in some cells. This results in a lowered autophagy process in association with protein. Progesterone and estrogen play a role in lowering the autophagy's basal levels in this instance. Women with diseases like polycystic ovary syndrome also show an increased likelihood of insulin resistance and overactive mTOR. There are also a host of other indicators and aspects that reveal the increased risk for women over men. The pathology for Alzheimer's can appear early in a child's life, revealing how there is a large difference in gender and the risk and severity of the disease. When mTOR is overly active, it causes the body to resist insulin. This activation can because by the presence of aggregated proteins, which glia and neurons cannot remove due to autophagy's low basal levels. When a body is stressed, it is good to slightly depress autophagy to help improve cell survival rates, but long-term and increased suppression leads to long-term illness.

The progression and even developing of Alzheimer's can be different in respect to the process of autophagy in men than in women. More studies are recommended to further examine the role of autophagy, age, and sex in Alzheimer's disease. These recommended additional studies will help scientists and doctors better understand the disease's pathology and ideal therapies for different genders.

Study #3: Genetic and Histological Evidence for Autophagy in Asthma Pathogenesis.

Link: https://www.jacionline.org/article/S0091-6749(11)01558-2/fulltext

Citation: "Genetic and histologic evidence for autophagy in asthma pathogenesis. Poon, Audrey H. et al. Journal of Allergy and Clinical Immunology, Volume 129, Issue 2, 569 – 571."

Asthma and the process of autophagy were never scientifically examined before the publication of this particular study. While it does not directly delineate between men and women in the study, it is a great example of the wide application and understanding of the importance of the autophagy process in the body. The findings of this study revealed that the formation of the autophagosome is elongated when ATG5 is included. The outer autophagosome membrane is formed by a complex combination of ATG16L1, ATG12, and ATG5. The risk of developing severe asthma can be related to the negative relationship between the allele "G" and the prebronchodilator "FEV". When the allele "G" is present, the patient is more likely to develop moderate or severe asthma. Asthmatic patients who suffer from poor lung function and moderate or severe asthma typically show tissue cells, specifically epithelial cells, and fibroblasts contain autophagosomes, which is genetically connected to prebronchodilator "FEV" and ATG5. While this study does not conclusively identify the part of autophagy and asthma, it presents a new perspective and avenue to explore. It provides a good example of the power and function of autophagy in multiple parts and functions of the body.

Chapter 8: Intermittent Fasting for Women

What is interesting to observe is how human eating patterns have changed over the years. It is also interesting to see how nutritional advice has changed. It seems like for many years, people began eating more, faster, and with meal times closer together. Nutritionists, fitness experts, and even doctors have also misunderstood science and results to promote unhealthy eating habits, like cutting out fat from the diet, increasing carbs, and eating frequent small meals. What we are now learning is that the "natural" way our bodies want to eat is actually better for optimal function and health. You are not designed to eat meals close to one another, consuming foods filled with chemicals. Actually, from an evolutionary standpoint, your body is more aligned with the survival needs of ancestors in the Paleolithic era, or about 10,000 BCE. This was a time of hunting and gathering for sustenance and also carried a strong uncertainty if food will be plentiful or scarce in the future. Sometimes, people would go through periods of "feasting" followed by lengths of "famine".

When you recognize that this is your natural, physiological, and biological design, you will be able to understand why it is important to "take a break" from eating every now and then. This is what brings your body into balance, including your hormones, brain, and digestion process. Cancer, obesity, autoimmune disease, heart disease, and diabetes all occur when the body's hormonal levels are unbalanced. With the current research being conducted and published, it is becoming more obvious every day that intermittent fasting can provide the tools for not just preventing, but treating diseases as well.

Your body and your preference determine what kind of intermittent fast is best for your health. It is also important to choose your type of intermittent fast based on your goals such as weight loss. But no matter what intermittent fasting method you choose, your hormones will be impacted. The major hormones that are affected include:

- Insulin
- Human Growth Hormone
- Leptin

- Ghrelin
- Estrogen
- Progesterone
- Cortisol
- Thyroid hormones

While intermittent fasting is one of the most exciting tools in health management and weight loss, there are some things you need to be careful with. Keeping your hormones in balance is one of those considerations. Sometimes, when you have illnesses cause by hormonal imbalance before starting, you should exercise extra caution. But, on the other hand, these people are probably some of the best candidates for intermittent fasting! This would be a great time to meet with your doctor to learn more about your options and use their guidance during the process.

Insulin is one of the most common hormones impacted while intermittent fasting. It is one of the hormones that actually seems to react to intermittent fasting the fastest and best. Many studies on animals showed that insulin levels stabilized; but now that there are a few human trials that have been published, it is evident that the majority of participants improved their sensitivity to insulin. When insulin rises after consuming glucose, the body participates in a series of responses. One of those responses is to support the absorption of glucose from the blood through the muscles, skeletal tissue, fat tissues, and liver. When that process is done, the liver then begins hoarding insulin as glycogen and then fat. As you continue to spike insulin levels, the body eventually becomes resistant to it. This resistance leads to inflammation and excessive fat stores. During intermittent fasting, you give your body a reprieve from the constant spiking of glucose. This allows your body to return, continue, or become sensitive to insulin.

Human Growth Hormone, or HGH, is another one that is dramatically improved with intermittent fasting, sometimes nicknamed the "fountain of youth" hormone. It is what protects and maintains your bone density and muscles. It is also what encourages the body to gather its energy from fat storage. It helps you look and feel better, too. When it is used synthetically, such as by athletes, it can also build muscles and improve physical performance. As you age, your HGH production reduces. To stimulate production, you can practice intermittent fasting. If you really want to boost HGH production, try fasting for a 5-day span. This has been shown to over double your HGH production! Of course, that can be tricky.

The place that intermittent fasting really shines for people looking to improve their metabolism is in the improvement of hormones linked to storing fat and interpreting hunger signals. Gherlin is nicknamed the "hunger" hormone. This little chemical's production changes positively during intermittent fasting. It is also interesting to note that improving gherlin production also improves dopamine production in the brain. This, in turn, enhances the function of the brain. This is a great example of the link between the digestive functions of the body and the brain. Another hormonal benefit during intermittent fasting is stabilizing leptins. Leptin resistance can cause stubborn weight gain and retention for many people. When you improve leptin sensitivity, you can begin to chip away at those stubborn pounds.

Of course, these are hormones men and women both have, but there are a few that are specific to just to women who are impacted during intermittent fasting. There is a specific path in your body where the brain talks directly to your ovaries. This is called the "hypothalamic-pituitary-gonadal" or the "brain-ovary axis". The ovaries respond to hormonal messages from the brain. These messages are what tells your ovaries to release progesterone and estrogen. When this axis is functioning properly, you can become pregnant. One of the reasons women are more receptive to the benefits of intermittent fasting than men is a chemical called kisspeptin. This is what makes women more "sensitive" to certain physical actions, such as fasting. Women typically have more kisspeptins than men. Because women are more sensitive due to more kisspeptins, they can also have disruption to their brain-ovary axis. This can result in irregular menstrual cycles and even skipped periods. Theoretically, it can also impact metabolism and fertility. More studies need to be conducted on this relationship and effect.

While intermittent fasting can disrupt hormonal levels, it can also improve them. It just depends on your body. For those that show to be sensitive to intermittent fasting, it is wise to begin gently and then build up as tolerance and body adjustments are improved.

Just above your kidneys, like little hats, sit your adrenal glands. These little "hats" secrete cortisol, which is the main hormone created when you are stressed. When the balance of your adrenal glands and your brain get unsettled, you suffer from a condition called "adrenal fatigue". This causes cortisol levels to increase when they should be low, lower when they should be high, or constantly high or low. This means that there is a host of dysfunctions that can occur in your adrenal glands. Another important hormone affected during intermittent fasting is the thyroid hormones, T3 and T4. These hormones impact every individual cell in the body. This means that if there is a thyroid dysfunction, your entire body will dysfunction. There are many reasons for thyroid hormonal disruptions a person can suffer from throughout your life. One issue is called Hashimoto's disease, an autoimmune problem. Another is T3 Syndrome, which is a problem with hormone conversion in the thyroid. You can also have a resistance built up to your thyroid hormones, similar to insulin resistance. There are also thyroid issues that occur when there is a problem with the pathway from the brain to the thyroid. If you suffer from a thyroid problem such as one of the ones mentioned above, you could respond differently to intermittent fasting than others.

Many people suffer from hormone imbalance in their life. It can occur in any pathway in the body and can interfere with the success of intermittent fasting but also can respond positively to it. If you suspect or know that your hormones are not balanced, make sure to begin slowly and gently into an intermittent plan, paying close attention to your body as you adjust or increase your eating plan.

There are certain steps you can take to help your hormone balance, not make it worse and also avoid feeling like you are hungry all the time. Sometimes, it can be challenging to find a good starting point. That is normal and okay! Be kind to yourself as you get going. If you choose a plan to start with and have a lot of trouble sticking to it or notice your body is going on a roller coaster ride of hormones, consider making an adjustment for the next time you are fasting. Maybe, it is fewer hours or more calories. If you decided to approach intermittent fasting aggressively and then binge eat the minute your fasting time is done, rolling on an emotional and energetic wave, consider cutting back to fewer days during the week or times during the day. You can always adjust until you find a place that is a challenge but still doable. And always celebrate your little wins. If you planned on fasting for 16 hours but broke your fast early at 12, take that as a win! It may not have been your ultimate goal, but 12 hours is a huge accomplishment! Same goes for if you cut down calories by 5% instead of 20%. That is still a good place to begin from and should be considered a success.

Women can thrive on an intermittent fasting regimen, but it will need to be supporting your hormonal balance, not disrupting it. This is especially important if you're beginning an intermittent fasting lifestyle within a healthy weight range. Your body, as a woman, can enter into a state of ketosis quicker than men, probably because of the kisspeptins, but it is also what makes your body more sensitive the feeling of being "hungry". A natural response in the female body when it feels like it is hungry is to make it feel and respond like it is starving. This can be heightened when you have a period of fasting and then introduce food again. The body ramps up production of gherlin and leptin, making you feel more hungry than you really are.

The important take away here is that for women, intermittent fasting can be an excellent method for losing weight, keeping it off, and supporting overall health; but it can also be harsh and uncomfortable if not approached mindfully. This is why it is important as a woman to be conscious of the fasting plan you have chosen, the plan for implementing it successfully into your life, and then listen to your body while you participate in your plan. Try to stick out the two-week introductory period to see if your body adjusts, but only if you are mildly uncomfortable, not disrupting or stressing your body unnecessarily. Stress unravels the success you can achieve when following an intermittent fasting plan, so find that special spot that is on the edge of your comfort zone, without causing distress. When you acclimate to this plan, then play around with increasing intensity. As a female, this is important for long-term success, hormonal balance, and overall health.

Chapter 9: How to Start Intermittent Fasting

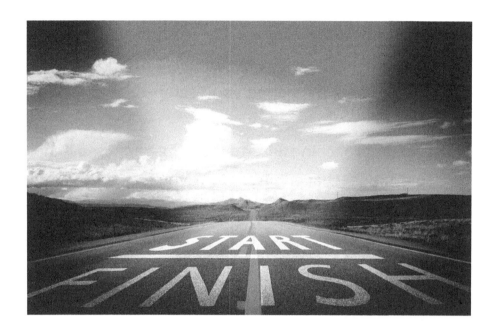

It can be a little overwhelming and intimidating to begin seriously considering and planning for intermittent fasting. It can also be discouraging when you see things splashed on social media like "Not even hungry on day 2 of my fast" or "Get fat adapted and you can make it three days without pain", and you are only a few hours in on your first day and are ravenous. When you feel like you have failed because you have cravings, broke your fast early or do not even start because you do not think you will succeed. You are not alone! So many people have been in your same shoes, you just may not see the filtered image and curated comments that highlight that part of intermittent fasting. It is not the "flashy" side. But there is a way that you can get started in your plan with confidence and ease. You have the ability to do it already, you may just need to change your perspective a little bit.

Instead of approaching intermittent fasting as a "chore" and something "challenging" that you have to "suffer" through, what if you considered as an "experiment" and something you are "exploring"? Set a realistic goal and let yourself to be curious about how your body will respond as you work towards that goal. Was your original starting point too aggressive for you? That is great! Now you know how to adjust for the next time. Did you make an adjustment to your starting point that was more successful? Awesome! Did you still struggle? What great new information you can use to adjust more favorably for your unique body? Keep watching what happens before, during, and after your fasting days. Analyze how you did and plan to make adjustments for the next time that you think will support you better. Constantly tweak and move forward. Just don't give up!

Also, consider your goal as a place to work towards and come up with a loose plan to achieve it. Do not create rigid restrictions that you feel you "must" follow to achieve your goal. Instead, choose a starting point that you feel aligns well with your short-term goal, and then give yourself a span of four weeks to find steps to work up to that goal. If you make it before four weeks, that is a win worth celebrating! If you take longer than four weeks to accomplish your goal, that is also a win worth celebrating! Four weeks is a guide. Sometimes, you will crush it, and other times, you will slide into another date. This is your body and your journey. No one has a biological or anatomical combination like you do. This means that you need to be mindful and gracious to your process.

Finally, do not tell yourself that this is a life-long, long-term commitment. It is a learning process to better support and understands your body. To learn about your body and your health, you get to experiment with it and learn about it while "doing". "Doing" in this instance is intermittent fasting. You do not need to feel boxed in and restricted from the joys of food and life! After all, this is one of the few eating plans that actually allows you to eat whatever you want! It is just experimenting with when you will eat these things and when you will not. Learn about when your body can do without and when it desires or needs something. The best way to experiment and learn this though is by giving is a shot.

Before you start your intermittent fasting process, you should consider a few things. Below is a little checklist to help you get set up in the right way:

- Discuss your plans with your medical doctors and team. If you have any medical condition or concern, this is absolutely essential! If at any point in the process you feel ill or disconnected, break your fast.

- Embrace the idea of keeping your plan simple. If the idea of counting calories and monitoring caloric intake is overwhelming, do not do it! Figure out how to easily introduce and maintain your plan.

- Do not forget to keep it easy, too. Do not disrupt your whole day for your fast. Try to keep things pretty much the same as during your "feasting" days. You can work on adjusting your nutritional intake on feast days if you are up for it, otherwise, pop a few good vitamins and get yourself acclimated to your plan first before adding more steps to the process. Sometimes, your goal is simply to start and finish a fast of any length. Do not confuse it with added or little goals that distract you from your first win.

- Pick and move times around to fit in with your life. Throughout the book, you were given times, such as 7 PM or 8:30 AM. These are provided to you for help in planning and understanding the concept. These are not doctrines. Adjust your times to fit what you need. For example, if you know you are going to eat an early dinner, decide if you want to start your fast at 5:45 PM or if you are going to enjoy a snack a little later in the evening to start your fast around 7:35 PM. Do not box yourself into a time that does not fit or needs to be adjusted on the day of your fast. It is fine! Make it work for you.

- Choose your days with care but also keep it flexible. Weekdays tend to be more structured and convenient for fasting for many people, but sometimes, it does not always work out well. For example, you may have been planning on fasting on Tuesday, but when you got into the office, there was a surprise party planned at lunch for a co-worker at your favorite restaurant followed by cake and ice cream. You may not want to miss this! If this is the case, maybe you want to break your fast for Tuesday, enjoy the celebration, and choose to fast on Wednesday instead. This kind of in-the-moment adjustment happens all the time. You get to choose how you are going to handle it, either you keep going with your original plan or move your fasting day to another day during the week. Of course, the option is there to skip the fasting day altogether, but try not to do this if you can avoid it.

- Give yourself a few "get out of jail free" cards. This means to recognize that you will probably slip up. Sometimes, this is a big slip up and a little hiccup. And sometimes, it happens a lot, while other times, it hardly ever happens. Do not beat yourself up, but rather let yourself off the hook and decide how you are going to get back on the plan. Maybe you start from the beginning again or maybe you just go to bed and start again the next day where you left off.

To help you get started with intermittent fasting even better, you need to have a clear purpose in mind. Be honest with yourself about the "why". Why do you want to do this? Is it for weight loss? Is it to improve your general health? Is it to help prevent various diseases, like cancer or neuro-degeneration? Once you get your answer, fill in a few blanks. For example, if you want to lose weight, how much weight are you looking to lose? Are hoping to remove daily or frequent medication for an illness? What do you take the medication for? Will your illness be impacted by your diet and how? If you want to prevent disease, which disease or diseases are you concerned about in particular? Why are you worried about these? Is it because the diseases are hereditary in your family or is it something you have been told you could develop later on? Being honest and clear about why you want to be in this kind of diet plan can not only help guide your goal-setting but also can be a motivational force keeping you on track. When things get uncomfortable, remember your purpose.

Now, take a moment to think about your concerns with intermittent fasting. What makes you most nervous about trying and sticking to your plan? This could be a serious concern or something less major. It does not matter how big or small your concern is. Take time to acknowledge and address it. Some of the most common concerns are actually tied to societal messaging that you hear often, such as "never miss breakfast for it is the most important meal of the day" or "you need to eat every few hours to keep your metabolism functioning". Intermittent fasting denies these norms and therefore can make people uneasy. To help you, it is good to look at the research behind the concern and behind intermittent fasting. For example, eating breakfast is not a "magic" plan. Skipping it does not mean you will have to gain weight or keep unwanted pounds on. It also does not mean your metabolism will be "jumpstarted" for the day if you eat it, and it does not mean you will have a sluggish metabolism if you skip it. Remember, the lengthy amount of research published on intermittent fasting shows that the best way to boot your metabolism and lose weight is through fat burning brought on with fasting. Another common concern is that you will lose muscle mass while fasting. Again, if this is your concern, you need to review the research published on how your body transitions from glucose to ketones for fuel. Ketones do not generate from your muscles, so your body is not breaking down muscle mass to keep you going, it is using your fat stores instead. If you are worried about your underlying health problems, set up an appointment to talk with your doctor about your intermittent fasting plan and what they think it will do for your body. Make sure to go prepared with your research to discuss key points with them to make sure your plan is setting you up for success.

When you begin your intermittent fasting plan, fall back to the old Chinese motto, "The temptation to quit will be greatest just before you are about to succeed." When you are feeling tempted to break your fast, drink a glass of water and distract yourself for 5 minutes. If the temptation is still there, get up and go for a 10-minute walk. Keep reminding yourself of your purpose and the Chinese proverb. Also, find ways to prevent yourself from reaching for after-dinner snacks. Your normal habits may include snuggling up on the couch and watching TV, along with a bowl of popcorn or ice cream. Instead, try a hot cup of herbal tea. You can also make sure to brush your teeth right after dinner. The taste is a known appetite suppressant, but it is also a mental message that you are no longer going to be eating for the day. It is also a good idea to go to bed early on a fasting night. Your body will suppress your cravings and hunger sensations while you sleep.

When you wake up in the morning, consider putting off your breakfast for a while. Do not grab something in a rush just "because", but rather enjoy a hot cup of coffee (with no milk or sugar) or tea until you have time to sit down and enjoy a meal. Breakfast doesn't need to be a rushed meal or something you "sneak" into your day. Instead, plan your day out and enjoy your breakfast after the rush has ended. This might mean you end up delaying your lunchtime, too. With just this one choice, you could be already moving your fasting window between late morning and nighttime, for example, 10 AM to 7 PM. After you make an adjustment like this, then you can look at adding in a few more steps, such as no more afternoon snacking.

Below are some aides to help you get through the mid-afternoon snacking impulse:

1. Remember that dinner is coming up soon. Remind yourself that food is coming and you are not starving. Give yourself permission to wait until dinnertime.

2. Time actually subsides the hunger impulse, not worsen it. If you find yourself feeling hungry, drink a cup of water and give yourself a time frame to "ride the wave" of hunger until it goes away.

3. This brings up another important tip: "hunger" can actually be thirst. And if it is not thirst, it could be a habit. It could also be emotional. There are many reasons your body feels "hungry" when it needs something else. Drinking a cup of water is always a safe way to test what you are really feeling. If it is a habit, try to break this habit by doing something else instead, like getting up for a walk around the office or making a cup of coffee. If you are responding to emotion, like stress or anger, find another way to work through emotions like physical exercise or meditation.

Chapter 10: Common Mistakes While Fasting and How to Avoid Them

One of the most common problems that people face with intermittent fasting is the immense amount of choice and flexibility it offers people. There are so many ways to do it that it leaves the opportunity for "mistakes" wide open. You choose an eating method that works for your life, but sometimes leads to problems. When you decide to try out intermittent fasting, no matter what method you choose or how you aim to do it, a few common mistakes are made often. One of the most common problems is giving up too soon. Others do not regulate their "feasting" meals properly, eating too much or too little when they have the opportunity or not eating "good" foods. Some people fall into the trap of going in too aggressively and trying to push their body to the limit. There are other common mistakes that occur, but no matter what happens, always remember that you can start back at the beginning if you need to!

The most common mistake people make when beginning and sticking to an intermittent fast is giving up early in the process. It is not easy. There will be times when it is uncomfortable. No matter what style of intermittent fasting you choose, it consists of reducing what you eat, breaking your habits, and making different choices. All of this is hard and difficult. You need discipline and commitment. And these traits need to be strong when the hunger hits. Keep in mind that as your body adapts to your new eating style, you will experience "growing" or "adjusting" pains. You may feel irritable and fatigued the first week or two, but once your nobody adjusts, you will notice less and less of this. So, when you are dragging your feet to bed early one night, mumbling to yourself about how ridiculous this is and you should just have that chocolate bar in the pantry, remember that this is going to pass and pass soon. And if you give it two or three weeks and the feelings are still there, then dial back the plan for now. It is possible that the method and structure you have chosen doesn't suit you where you are at right now. Back off a bit, give your body a break and try a new approach. Just don't give up! Keep working towards your goals. You can do this!

The food you consume on your feasting days is another common mistake. Now, there is a caveat here. Many times, when you begin intermittent fasting, you are just focused on completing a fast, not on the food you are eating on a feast day. But if you have seen success for a few weeks, then it's time for you to start examining how you eat during those non-fasting moments. When you start looking into your caloric consumption and the nutritional components for your meals, you may find yourself falling into one of the common "mistake" categories: eating too much, not eating enough, or eating the "wrong" foods. When you break a fast, especially in the beginning, your body may be sending some pretty powerful messages that you need to eat, right now, anything and everything you can get your hands on. You may find yourself consuming your entire days' worth of calories in just one sitting! In the beginning, do not worry too much about this unless it makes you ill and uncomfortable. Instead, celebrate your win of the fast and worry about your food later. When "later" comes, however, you need to take a look at your habits. Ideally, you want to catch your "mistakes" with food early so they do not become something hard to break, but rather a small tweak or adjustment. People looking to lose weight will find it hard to see the big gains they want if they are eating too much when they break their fast. If you are willing to wait to see the pounds slide off, this is good, but it can be very unmotivating for many. Instead, making sure you do not overeat on your feasting days is critical to helping you lose the weight and keep it off.

It is common to find yourself in a situation where your "eyes are bigger than your stomach", meaning that your body feels that it is so hungry it needs much more than it can physically hold. Remember, losing weight is about bringing in fewer calories than you are putting out. To help make sure you get this, try planning and portioning out your meals ahead of time. This way it is a "grab-and-go" type of situation, with the "right" amount of calories for your normal life.

You can manually track what you eat as well. Watching the nutrients and calories of the foods and drinks you are consuming provides powerful information about your progress towards your goals. If you do not want to keep a paper journal of your meals, consider an online resource or app to support you. This way you know exactly how your intake is stacking up against your output. This resource also helps you recognize where you need to cut back on and where you need to beef up for optimal health and weight benefits.

In addition, when you sit down to eat, give yourself time to savor your meal. Try starting the meal off with a glass of water, and then pause between bites and courses, if applicable. It takes time for your body to recognize it is full. If you begin shoveling down the food as soon as you sit down, you deny your brain the time to read the messages from the stomach. Give yourself the time to listen to your body so you can tell the difference between wanting more and needing more.

The other side of the coin are the people that continue their fast when they are supposed to break it. The idea many explain is that they do not want to "undo" what they had done during their non-eating period. People may also think that if they eat too much, the next fast will be harder to accomplish. The problem with this is that your body moves from ketosis to starvation ketosis this way. If you deny your body the nutrients it needs to function properly, eventually, it runs out of fat storage and goes into true "emergency" mode. When you get into this state, your metabolism slows down so much it can almost appear to be stopped. Now, you went from burning fat for fuel to storing it up again. Remember that your body needs a good amount of food—it is called a "feast" day for a reason! Without enough sustenance your body will not function properly, your brain will become cloudy, and you will not have the same "personality" as you did when you had nutrition coming in.

It is normal to feel irritable, weak, tired, and cloudy when you are fasting, but when you reintroduce food, you should see those symptoms dissipate. If they persist, chances are you are not giving your body enough calories. Like overeating, undereaters can benefit from tracking their food and drink intake to identify the areas that they need to ramp up or cut back on. For example, eating a lot of junk food and not enough whole foods can rob your body of the nutrients it needs. A manual food journal or an online resource or application is a great way to make sure you get what you need.

This leads to the third part of food mistakes: choosing to eat the "wrong" foods. When you stop eating food all the time, the food you eat becomes that much more important. This goes beyond just counting your calories.

Now, you are diving into the nutrients of food and your dietary needs, and you are starting to find foods within your calorie range but also pack the most nutrients in. A great example is an avocado. It has 500 calories, but the nutrition it provides to the body, such as a good source of "healthy" fat, is a much better choice for your body than a processed bag of pretzels that is also 500 calories. Same calories, much different impact on your body! When you are ready to start diving into your nutrition, this is a great place to examine and refine. Fill your meals and snacks on feasting days with good carbs, lean protein sources, and healthy fats. Choose whole foods over processed ones. And do not forget fiber! This is a great addition that helps with digestion, including bloating and gas. If you can choose mostly healthy foods for your meals and non-fasting days, you help support your body's overall health and weight goals better than ignoring what you put in your mouth. But that being said, enjoying a warm chocolate chip cookie or a salty snack every now and then is not the end of the world!

And, while on the subject of healthy choices, make sure you always have water handy. If you are sick or bored of still water, swap it out for sparkling water or toss some fresh fruit in there to flavor it up. And you also do not need to only drink water while fasting. No, you cannot have a latte or a double chocolate frappuccino with extra drizzle and extra whip with extra everything else. But you can have a good, hot cup of black coffee or herbal tea. You do not want to add anything to it that will introduce calories into your fast, but you can sip on something flavorful, which can often trick your brain into thinking it has gotten its wanted sustenance. In addition, the mind often mixes up the signal for thirst with the signal for hunger. What you may be feeling is not really hunger, but you are thirsty and need water. The more you drink during a fasting day, the better you will do and the better you will feel. A good idea is to invest in a pretty and functional water bottle that you can take around with you all the time. Keep filling it up when it gets low or empty and make sure you sip on it regularly. If you really need to, set reminders on your phone or alarms for times of the day to keep you drinking often. If you ever experience a fasting day with little water and then compare it to fasting days when you had good hydration, you will notice a dramatic difference in your experience. Hopefully, you will just trust this and not try that out for yourself!

Intermittent fasting is not starvation. These are two different phases of food consumption, although your mind may not always recognize it when you are hungry on your fasting day. The reality, however, is you need food to survive. When you take away food too much, you negatively impact your life, which is the opposite of the intention behind intermittent fasting. Fasting mimics the evolutionary wiring in the brain that dates back to the Paleolithic era; it is a healthy and natural process. Starvation is not. This means your body starts to shut down, including your brain. If you find yourself pushing your fast to be longer, more frequent, and with less and less food, you will probably start to notice continual problems with your everyday functioning. You are also probably entering into disorder "territory". You do not need to overdo it. Find a good place to rest that is sustainable for the long-term and that supports your health goals and healthy weight. Do not fall into this trap of pushing too hard and too far. It is about balance and health, not a competition who can live the longest without eating food. No one wins that competition.

Finally, the last mistake almost all people face, no matter the method of Intermittent fasting chosen, is trying to fit a "square peg in a round hole". What this means is that if you are absolutely miserable and ridiculous while fasting and cannot find a suitable plan that fits your life, do not try to force it into your lifestyle. It is not always the best solution for everyone. Sometimes, it is your plan or the process or adapting to fat burning; sometimes, it is just your body composition. You may have a health issue that does not do well with fasting, like type 1 diabetes, or maybe your lifestyle does not allow or need for caloric restrictions, such as extremely active athletes and physical fitness experts. These people may need a constant supply of energy because their body does not have a lot of stored fat, and they are constantly using their incoming energy. Yes, intermittent fasting reinforces the way most bodies are designed to eat, but not all bodies are the same, and there have been a "few" environmental changes to our world since the Paleolithic era that can also impact your ability to fast.

In some traditions, people are designated into different body types that respond to fasting in different ways. For example, in the Ayurvedic tradition, there are three different types of people. The Kaphic body is more suitable to skipping breakfast, but tends to hold on to fat more and can have a sluggish metabolism. On the other hand, a Vata body has a more flighty meal pattern naturally, making it easy to fast sometimes and disorientating other times. The third body type, Pitta, usually have strong digestion and metabolism, requiring a constant supply of food for energy. This means fasting could throw their natural body functions off balance instead of supporting it. In addition, Pittas tend to be very competitive, turning a standard intermittent fast into a competition. And like mentioned above, this is not always a good thing when dealing with the fuel source for proper body function.

Intermittent fasting should bring balance and health to your life. If you find that you are just miserable every time you "have" to fast, it is okay to ask yourself if the benefits of the fast are greater than the quality of life and happiness you are sacrificing. If you find that the misery is greater than the results, maybe you should rethink your approach to intermittent fasting altogether. There are other diet plans out there that may be better suited for your success.

Recall back to when you shifted your perspective from "have" to do intermittent fasting, despite how "hard" and "difficult" it is, to a fresh view of a new experiment designed to teach you about yourself and your body. When you find yourself struggling with one of these "mistakes" or one of the myriads of other "mistakes" you can encounter with such a broad approach to eating, bring your mindset back to one of curiosity and learning. Give yourself permission to experiment with what works and what does not without stamping a big "F" on your efforts. Even if you decide that intermittent fasting is not for you, you deserve a gold star and a celebration for taking the time to learn more about your body and its needs. That is a huge win and accomplishment you should embrace!

Conclusion

Thanks for making it through to the end of *Intermittent Fasting for Women: The Complete Beginner's Guide for Weight Loss—Burn Fat, Heal Your Body Through the Special Intermittent Process, and Live a Healthy Lifestyle.* Let's hope it was informative and able to provide you with all of the tools you need to achieve your goals whatever they may be.

Now that you have finished learning about it, the next step you need to take it to decide how you are going to take action. It is not enough to think about it. Now you need to apply what you have read so you can continue to learn through doing it. Through this application, you have the ability to influence your mental state, your waistline, the number popping up on the scale, and your general health. That is very impactful and empowering! But you have to get started. You probably already have an idea of how you would fit this into your life. If not, head back to Chapters 3 and 9 to revisit some methods for applying it to your life. This way, when you dip your toes in or dive head first into intermittent fasting, you will have a good idea of how it will go so you can be confident in your decisions. The idea is to create a life-long change to how you approach your caloric intake, but it is flexible and adaptable. In the beginning, you will want to experiment and explore what will work for you. Do not fall into the trap of feeling like you "failed" because things did not go according to your plan. Instead, find something worth celebrating; even reading this book is something worth celebrating because you are now that much closer!

Keep moving forward on your journey to improve your health and waistline! You can do it!

Finally, if you found this book useful in any way, a review on Amazon is always appreciated!

Thank You !

Made in the USA
Middletown, DE
28 August 2019